Practical Sonography
in
Obstetrics and Gynecology

Second Edition

Practical Sonography in Obstetrics and Gynecology

Second Edition

John W. Seeds, M.D.
Vice Chair and Professor
Department of Obstetrics and Gynecology
Division of Maternal-Fetal Medicine
Virginia Commonwealth University
Medical College of Virginia
School of Medicine
Richmond, Virginia

Nancy C. Chescheir, M.D.
Associate Professor
Division of Maternal-Fetal Medicine
Department of Obstetrics and Gynecology
University of North Carolina
Chapel Hill, North Carolina

Ronald V. Wade, M.D.
Vice President for Medical Education and Chairman
Department of Obstetrics and Gynecology
Medical Director, Women's Institute
Carolinas Medical Center
Charlotte, North Carolina

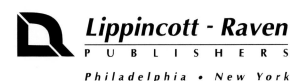

Lippincott - Raven
P U B L I S H E R S

Philadelphia • New York

Lippincott-Raven Publishers, 227 East Washington Square, Philadelphia, Pennsylvania 19106

Made in the United States of America

Library of Congress Cataloging-in-Publication Data

Seeds, John W.
    Practical sonography in obstetrics and gynecology / John W. Seeds,
Nancy C. Chescheir, Ronald V. Wade.--2nd ed.
        p.   cm.
    Rev. ed. of: Practical obstetrical ultrasound / John W. Seeds,
Robert C. Cefalo. 1986.
    Includes bibliographical references and index.
    ISBN 0-7817-0335-2
    1. Ultrasonics in obstetrics.   2. Generative organs, Female-
-Ultrasonic imaging.   I. Chescheir, Nancy.   II. Wade, Ronald V.
III. Seeds, John W. Practical obstetrical ultrasound.   IV. Title.
    [DNLM: 1. Ultrasonography, Prenatal.   2. Pregnancy Complications-
-ultrasonography.   3. Genital Diseases, Female--ultrasonography.
WQ 209 S451p 1996]
RG527.5.U48S44 1996
618´ .047543--dc20
DNLM/DLC
for Library of Congress   95-11323

9   8   7   6   5   4   3   2   1

To our patients
whose experiences with ultrasound
provide the basis for the illustrations
in this book.

J.W.S.

To those who have given me the opportunity to learn ultrasound:
my mentors,
the patients with whom I've had the honor of working,
the sonographers who have worked with me,
the learners who always prod me to learn more,
and to my parents.

N.C.C.

To the sonographers
and residents
I have had the privilege of teaching
and learning from
over the years.

R.V.W.

Contents

Preface

Since the introduction of realtime ultrasound in 1977, sonography has become an indispensible tool in the care of pregnancy and is becoming a valuable adjunct in the care of a wide variety of gynecologic problems.

Over the years, the equipment has steadily improved and our ability to use it has grown. Training in sonography is now included in the residency requirements in obstetrics and gynecology as well as in radiology, and certification board examinations in both specialties include questions about ultrasound. Postgraduate courses in ultrasound in obstetrics and gynecology are commonplace.

Issues regularly debated include: who should be performing obstetric and gynecologic ultrasound, which patients should undergo ultrasound examinations, how is appropriate reimbursement ensured, what specific components should be included in every examination, and how is liability determined. As our ability to detect ever more subtle fetal abnormalities has grown, the clinician's anxiety over possible missed diagnoses has increased.

We have tried to address each of these concerns in chapters that are practical, readable, and informative. Illustrations, both line art and sonograms, provide specific information intended to increase the reader's understanding. Specific guidelines for the appropriate content of an ultrasound examination are provided. The use of ultrasound in gestational dating and monitoring fetal growth is reviewed. The basis and technique for endovaginal ultrasound in both obstetrics and gynecology are presented. Ultrasound in the assessment of fetal well-being and specific guidelines for the diagnosis of fetal malformations are presented and illustrated. Finally, specific methods for minimizing medical liability through the performance and documentation of the best possible service are provided.

Whether or not the clinician providing obstetric and gynecologic care is personally involved in sonographic imaging, the information presented here is important for proper and defensible medical management. The appropriate use of sonographic information is as important as the actual performance of the exam, and knowledge of the technique is needed for both.

Therefore, sonographers, both radiologic and obstetric sonologists, and any clinician active in obstetrics and gynecology who uses ultrasound in the care of his or her patients, should be aware of the principles presented in this book.

Practical Sonography
in
Obstetrics and Gynecology

Second Edition

1

Basic Physics, Formatting, and Image Development

The image depicted on the screen of a modern ultrasound machine is not biologic reality; it is a visual simulation of biologic reality constructed from echoes detected at the surface of the patient. The physical nature of the echoes, the interaction of sound with tissue, and the manipulation of this information to produce visual images must be understood to some extent to properly interpret these images. Lack of understanding can lead to errors of diagnosis and even inappropriate interventions or inaccurate counseling. The minimal necessary understanding of the physical basis of ultrasound imaging is not difficult and is well within the grasp of any clinician interested in obstetric and gynecologic ultrasound. A review of this chapter is, therefore, strongly encouraged as a first step in the introduction to clinical ultrasound. The depth and detail of this discussion is meant to prepare the reader for the interpretation of images, but it is insufficient preparation for the physics portion of any technical registry examination.

SOUND

Sound is a form of **kinetic energy;** it is not electromagnetic or ionizing energy. Sound physically agitates the molecules of the propagation medium. As the surface of the sound source pushes molecules closer to their neighbors, the natural electromagnetic intermolecular forces defining the structural nature of that substance immediately begin to reestablish the normal intermolecular spatial relationships and, in doing so, transmit the energy of compression to the next adjacent spacial zone of the medium. It is this spring-like quality of the natural intermolecular forces that accepts, stores briefly, and then propagates the kinetic sound energy through any medium that is the basis for diagnostic ultrasound.

Sound is characterized by alternate phases of high and low pressure, or density, that follow a pattern of repetition. Any given sound may then be characterized by a specific frequency (expressed as complete cycles per second), by wavelength, or by amplitude. Sound is often referred to as "sound waves," but the

1

sound cycles are not really similar to waves on the surface of water. Sound is naturally three dimensional, as is most radiant energy, and, although sound simulates the shape and size of the source for a limited time or distance, this spatial molecular distortion we call *sound* typically spreads in all directions (divergence) eventually as it dissipates.

Kinetic sound energy is continuously transformed into thermal energy as it propagates through any medium. Therefore, any sound system has a definable and limited range of transmission from the source that depends on the intensity or power at the origin and on the rate of transformation to thermal energy or heat. Characteristics that influence the rate of transformation of sound energy to heat include frequency and impedance. The higher the frequency of the sound, the more rapidly the energy is transformed to heat, and the more limited is the transmission range. The higher the impedence of the medium, that is, the resistance of the intermolecular forces to distortion, the more rapidly the energy is dissipated as heat. Ultrasound energy, for instance, is rapidly dissipated in bone, and therefore, the temperature change at the surface of bone would be expected to be higher than the temperature change in soft tissue. Furthermore, any temperature change might be expected to be higher in higher frequency sound systems and the penetration, lower.

ULTRASOUND

Ultrasound is any sound system with a frequency over 20,000 cycles per second, or 20 kilohertz. This is the theoretical upper limit of hearing of the human ear. Medical applications typically involve sound frequencies between 1 and 10 million cycles per second, or 1–10 megahertz. Imaging systems in obstetrics and gynecology usually use frequencies between 3.5 and 7 megahertz. Imaging applications concerned with more superficial structures, such as peripheral vascular uses interested in superficial arterial structures may find systems up to 10 megahertz useful.

PIEZOELECTRIC CRYSTALS

Imaging systems use intermittent pulses of high frequency sound. The production of sound pulses of millions of cycles per second requires piezoelectric crystals. Piezoelectric crystals demonstrate the unique natural property of changing their shape when exposed to brief pulses of electric potential (Fig. 1-1). After a brief electronic pulse, these crystals continue to vibrate like guitar strings, with unique frequencies determined by shape, size, thickness, and crystalline structure. Quartz is a naturally occurring piezoelectric crystal. Modern ultrasound machines typically use synthetic piezoelectric crystals.

A critical property of the piezoelectric crystals is that they not only generate sound pulses of extraordinarily high frequency, but they can also detect such

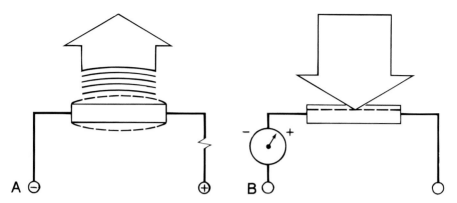

FIG. 1-1. The piezoelectric crystal demonstrates the dual property of generating sound of extremely high frequency when stimulated with electric potential **(A)**, and also generating a small electric potential when in the path of incoming sound pressure pulses **(B)**. [Source: Reprinted from *Practical Obstetrical Ultrasound* (p. 5) by J. W. Seeds and R. C. Cefalo, Aspen Publishers, Inc., Rockville, MD, © 1986.]

sound. When a piezoelectric crystal is squeezed, as it would be squeezed in the high-pressure phase of an incoming sound pulse or echo, the crystal generates a small electric potential. This potential may be detected, its intensity measured, and its time of detection catalogued. Such information forms the basis of measurement or imaging. The system is designed to use the time interval from transmission of the initial sound pulse to detection of echo as the basis for estimation of the distance from transducer surface to the surface that produced the echo.

TRANSDUCERS

Transducers are devices that convert (transduce) electronic energy to sound energy. The piezoelectric crystal is built into the surface of the device, usually with a damping substance behind it, like a shock absorber that prevents unwanted persistent vibration, and there must be a wire connecting the device to the electronic source or machine (Fig. 1-2).

The alternating phases of high and low pressure or molecular density that we call *sound*, emanating from the surface of this simple single crystal transducer will propagate through the adjacent medium and away from the transducer. The phases of molecular compression and rarefaction that constitute this "sound" system will maintain a reasonable fidelity to the shape and size of the originating crystal until divergence acts at the edges to expand the area affected (Fig. 1-3). The zone closest to the transducer, where the sound "beam" is the "tightest" is where such a sound system provides the most precise imaging or sharpest resolution. Divergence will inevitably diminish the intensity of the pulse and degrade the resolution of the image as distance from the transducer increases. Intensity is diminished since the total energy of the pulse is diluted over a larger area of

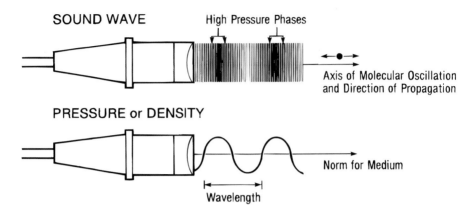

FIG. 1-2. The simple, single crystal transducer shown here generates a single beam of sound energy from its surface that may be described in terms of frequency, wavelength, and amplitude, based on characteristics of the repetitive sequenced phases of high and low pressure. [Source: Reprinted from *Practical Obstetrical Ultrasound* (p. 4) by J. W. Seeds and R. C. Cefalo, Aspen Publishers, Inc., Rockville, MD, © 1986.]

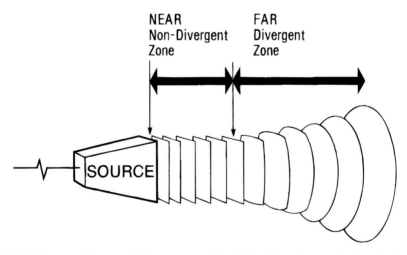

FIG. 1-3. The sound beam maintains a reasonable fidelity to the shape and size of the transducer until divergence begins at the edges to spread the energy of each energy phase over a broader area. Resolution suffers since points across the path of the sound beam will not be resolved as separate with a larger beamwidth that produces simultaneous echoes from the two points. [Source: Reprinted from *Practical Obstetrical Ultrasound* (p. 5) by J. W. Seeds and R. C. Cefalo, Aspen Publishers, Inc., Rockville, MD, © 1986.]

medium. Resolution is diminished since the larger size pulse will encounter more diverse points of anatomy simultaneously and the simultaneous echoes produced will be indistinguishable.

Pulse-Echo Principle

Continuous sound generation would result in continuous and confusing echo production. Therefore, ultrasound imaging systems generate discrete pulses of ultrasound and listen for discrete echoes . Pulse repetition frequency (PRF) can vary with different applications, but, for realtime imaging systems, typically, any given crystal is producing sound energy for a microsecond at millisecond intervals. In other words, a given crystal is active for only a tenth of one percent of any given time interval. Furthermore, since it may be estimated (based on an assumed speed of sound in soft tissue of about 1540 meters per second and a useful imaging depth of about 20 cm) that any real or true echo will have returned in about one quarter of this interval, systems may be designed to ignore noise heard during a majority of the inactive interval.

Linear Ranging

Sound pulses and echoes may be used for linear ranging or for imaging. If you know when a primary pulse was generated, when an echo was heard, and what the speed of sound in that medium is, you can calculate the distance of the echo-generating object from the transducer (linear ranging). This is the principle basis of imaging and was the basis for the early uses of ultrasound, often called *A-mode* ultrasound (Fig. 1-4). The speed of sound in soft tissue is set by convention to be

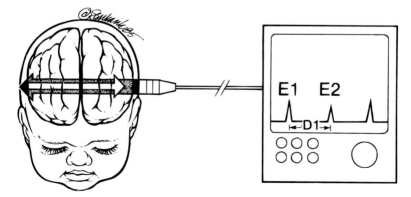

FIG. 1-4. A-mode ultrasound used a single crystal to produce pulses and to listen for echoes at a single point. The echoes then modulated the baseline of an oscilliscope (amplitude modulation, hence A-mode). If calibrated for the speed of sound, the distance between spikes could be measured, and the distance between the transducer surface and the tissue surface producing the echo could be estimated (linear ranging). [Source: Reprinted from *Practical Obstetrical Ultrasound* (p. 8) by J. W. Seeds and R. C. Cefalo, Aspen Publishers, Inc., Rockville, MD, © 1986.]

1540 m/sec, although this specific speed is exactly true for only a few limited tissues. A computer tracks the time of generation, the time of echo reception, and catalogues the echoes heard.

TISSUE INTERACTION

Sound pulses traveling through soft tissue encounter tissue surfaces, or interfaces, between different tissues. At these surfaces, the sound pulse may be reflected, transmitted, or refracted (Fig. 1-5). If the two tissues at an interface are identical, the pulse is transmitted largely unchanged. If the two interfaced tissues differ in terms of **acoustical impedence** (intermolecular stiffness), an echo is generated. The intensity, or amplitude, of the echo is proportional to the acoustical impedance difference or mismatch between the two tissues. In any case, since energy is not created at the surface, the amplitude of any echo must be subtracted from the amplitude of the transmitted pulse. Therefore, imaging of complex tissues more rapidly depletes the available energy of an ultrasound system as the energy is used up by echoes. Conversely, a homogeneous medium (liquid in blad-

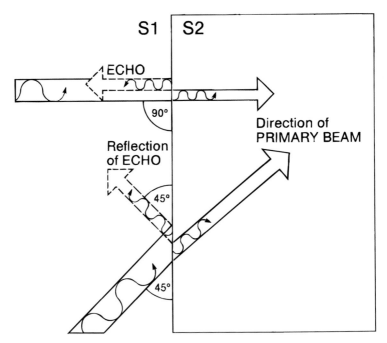

FIG. 1-5. Primary sound pulses encountering a surface between two tissues (S1 and S2) may be reflected as echoes or transmitted. The energy of an echo must be subtracted from the energy of the portion transmitted, hence, with complex tissues producing many echoes, the energy of the primary pulse is expended rapidly. Also note that only echoes from surfaces at a right angle to the direction of propagation will be detected at the transducer. Echoes at other angles are lost. [Source: Reprinted from *Practical Obstetrical Ultrasound* (p. 7) by J. W. Seeds and R. C. Cefalo, Aspen Publishers, Inc., Rockville, MD, © 1986.]

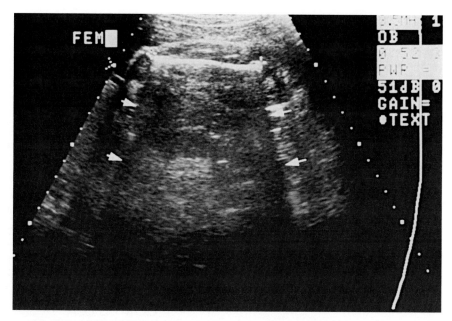

FIG. 1-6. This image of a fetal femur demonstrates **acoustic shadows** under the bone, since the majority of energy is reflected at the surface of the bone or dissipated in the relatively dense tissue of the bone. Deep in the image, to either side of the bone, **enhancement** of the tissue detail results from the increased **through transmission** of sound pulses through the amniotic fluid.

der, ovarian cyst, amniotic fluid) generates few echoes, results in **increased through transmission,** preserves more energy in the pulses, and results in **enhancement** of imaging of deeper tissues (Fig. 1-6).

The echoes generated at a tissue surface, or interface, will be detected by the appropriate crystal only if they encounter and are reflected by a surface positioned at 90 degrees to the **direction of propagation.** If the primary pulse encounters a surface at any angle other than 90 degrees, the echoes are scattered and lost, and that portion of the incoming pulse that is transmitted will be refracted at a slight angle to the original vector. These are relevant considerations when imaging the oval fetal cranium, for instance. Reflection of energy from curved surfaces and refraction of transmitted energy through those same curved surfaces typically produces a divergent anechoic area below the curvature where no anatomic information is provided. Failure to consider the possible contribution of refraction to this image may result in the inaccurate suspicion of a malformation.

STATIC GRAY SCALE

Early imaging machines mounted a single crystal transducer at the end of an electromechanical arm. Marking the starting point, the operator moves the transducer across the subject, while the machine generates a rapid sequence of successive sound pulses, listens for the echoes, and catalogues the estimated distances of the echoes as well as the exact position of the transducer relative to the starting point at the time an echo was detected (Fig. 1-7). This accumulated data allows the reconstruction of a composite image of anatomy based on this information. These machines were called variously "static," "B-scanners," "compound," "contact scanners," or "gray scale" machines.

"Static" referred to the fact that the images were necessarily motionless and developed one at a time. In fact, if any element of anatomy within the plane of the scan moved, the image was degraded by the movement. This feature complicated obstetric scanning whenever the fetus moved. **"B-scan"** was a term that arose from the fact that the reception of an echo resulted in the modulation of the brightness (**B** stood for brightness) of a spot (now more often called *pixel*) on the cathode ray tube (video screen). **"Compound"** was sometimes used since these scanners produced an image compounded from information from many echoes,

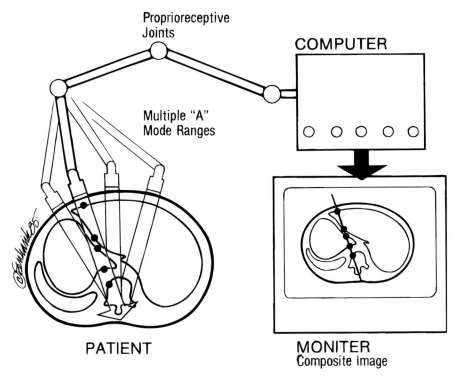

FIG. 1-7. Early **static** ultrasound imagers used a single crystal transducer moved in one plane in **contact** with the patient with accumulation of echo data and the construction of a **compound** image from the many echoes. Stillness of the subject was essential to clarity of image, since, if the subject moved, the geometric relationships would be lost. [Source: Reprinted from *Practical Obstetrical Ultrasound* (p. 9) by J. W. Seeds and R. C. Cefalo, Aspen Publishers, Inc., Rockville, MD, © 1986.]

and **"contact"** was occasionally used since the transducer actually touched the patient. Some older scanners used a transducer that moved across the surface of a waterbath in which the patient was immersed. Finally **"gray scale"** referred to a later development that adjusted the brightness of the spot on the video screen to correspond to the relative intensity of the echo producing that spot.

REALTIME LINEAR ARRAY

The next major development in ultrasound imaging was the **linear array realtime** ultrasound transducer. The manufacture and alignment of multiple crystal elements fixed to one another and rapidly activated in overlapping teams of four or five crystals in sequence across the length of the transducer produce complete rectangular images in a small fraction of a second (Fig. 1-8). The image displayed on the videoscreen is replaced with a new one up to 32 times a second and, therefore, movement in realtime may be shown. This design also allows

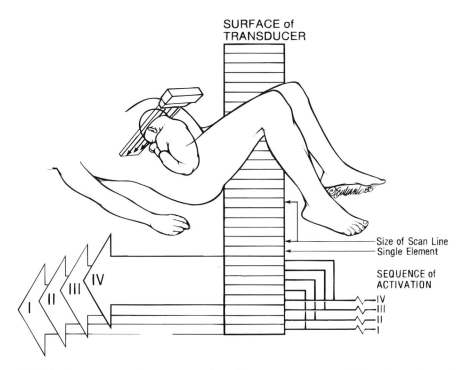

FIG. 1-8. Linear array, and convex array transducers use many crystals aligned together, and activated in teams to produce overlapping scanlines sequenced rapidly along the surface to produce images updated onscreen rapidly enough to eliminate visible frame changes, hence realtime movement. Since the crystals are aligned permanently, freehand movement is allowed. [Source: Reprinted from *Practical Obstetrical Ultrasound* (p. 10) by J. W. Seeds and R. C. Cefalo, Aspen Publishers, Inc., Rockville, MD, © 1986.]

the transducer to be moved freely in space without the need for any electro-mechanical arm, since the spatial relationships of the crystal teams are constant.

CONVEX ARRAY

Convex linear array (curvilinear) transducers have become popular because they are small, light, easily manipulated, and produce divergent images of deep anatomy from relatively small contact areas or apertures. These transducers are analogous in many ways to linear array transducers but are designed with a convex, or curved, contact surface that results in a divergent field of view or scanplane. Such a device can image a larger deep field with a relatively smaller contact surface and a physically smaller transducer that facilitates manipulation and handling. Furthermore, since the scanlines are radiating in a divergent pattern, reverberation artifacts that often complicate linear array images may be reduced with convex array imaging.

RESOLUTION

The sharpness of the visual image, or resolution, represents the ability of the device to discriminate adjacent points of anatomy as separate. The closer the points of anatomy that may be discriminated as separate, the better the resolution. Ultrasound resolution is defined in three planes that correspond to specific dimensions of the image.

Axial resolution is the ability to discriminate as separate two points aligned along the direction of propagation of the sound system. This is usually the vertical dimension of the displayed image. Axial resolution is influenced by and proportional to pulse length. The smaller the pulse, the better the axial resolution. Higher frequencies have shorter wavelengths and shorter pulses (Fig. 1-9). Higher frequency transducers, therefore, have better axial resolution, but their energy is used up faster, and they demonstrate diminished depth of penetration. Abdominal scanning that targets deep fetal anatomy in a near-term pregnancy in a heavy-set patient is best done with lower frequency transducers such as 2.5 or 3.5 megahertz, since the penetration is deeper with the lower frequency. First trimester endovaginal scanning in which the target is near the transducer located in a vaginal fornix may be done well with 7 megahertz scanners that provide exceptional resolution. Some manufacturers offer multiple frequency transducers that allow selection of frequency instead of changing transducers to suit unique applications.

Lateral resolution is the ability to discriminate two points aligned across the direction of propagation. This is usually the horizontal dimension of the displayed image. Lateral resolution is a function of beamwidth. Divergence increases beamwidth and damages lateral resolution. Two methods of minimizing beamwidth are used to maximize lateral resolution. First, the crystal may be man-

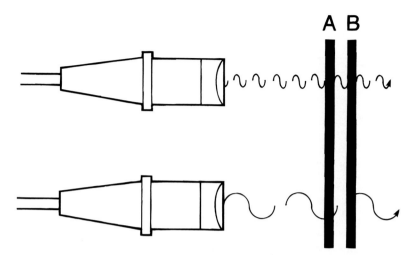

FIG. 1-9. The ability to discriminate surface A from surface B is described as axial resolution and is a function of pulse length. High frequencies allow shorter pulse length and improved axial resolution as shown here. [Source: Reprinted from *Practical Obstetrical Ultrasound* (p. 15) by J. W. Seeds and R. C. Cefalo, Aspen Publishers, Inc., Rockville, MD, © 1986.]

ufactured in a curved shape, focusing the beam to a minimum beamwidth at a specified depth of maximum resolution, but this focal length cannot be varied after manufacture (Fig. 1-10). Points of anatomy that are physically the same distance apart may be discriminated only at the depth of minimum beamwidth.

Another method for minimizing beamwidth is electronic focusing. The beam may be electronically focused by asynchronously pulsing the outside members of the crystal teams, forcing each pulse beam inward to a minimum beamwidth at a specified depth (Fig. 1-11). The focal length of the beam is a function of the de-

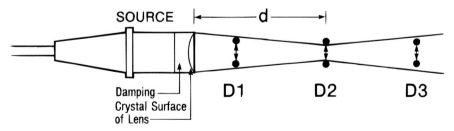

FIG. 1-10. Lateral resolution is a function of beamwidth, and deteriorates with divergence. One method of improved lateral resolution illustrated here is derived from manufacturing the crystal in a shape that focuses the pulse to a minimum beamwidth at a fixed depth, D2. At D1 and D3, points of anatomy an identical distance apart are not resolved, while at D2, these points may be resolved. [Source: Reprinted from *Practical Obstetrical Ultrasound* (p. 12) by J. W. Seeds and R. C. Cefalo, Aspen Publishers, Inc., Rockville, MD, © 1986.]

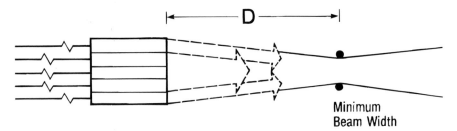

FIG. 1-11. Another method of minimizing beamwidth and maximizing lateral resolution is to activate the outboard members of a team of crystals slightly before the inner members, forcing the sound pulses to a minimum beamwidth at a given distance from the transducer. The asynchrony may be varied electronically, allowing some user control of the depth of best lateral resolution. [Source: Reprinted from *Practical Obstetrical Ultrasound* (p. 13) by J. W. Seeds and R. C. Cefalo, Aspen Publishers, Inc., Rockville, MD, © 1986.]

gree of asynchrony and may therefore be changed electronically. This is the basis for the focal zone adjustments on most machines.

In practice, both methods are used. The sound pulses from any team of crystals, though, is subject to divergence in the lateral dimension, but also in the **azimuthal plane,** the dimension perpendicular to the image slice, the thickness of the slice of anatomy.

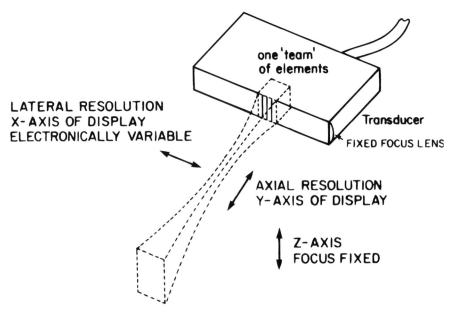

FIG. 1-12. Modern linear or convex transducers use all three methodologies to produce optimal images. Fixed focal depths are built in to control divergence in the azimuthal plane, while electronic focusing is used to vary focal zones in the horizontal dimension of the image, and frequency is used to produce an optimal compromise between image clarity and penetration. [Source: Reprinted from *Practical Obstetrical Ultrasound* (p. 14) by J. W. Seeds and R. C. Cefalo, Aspen Publishers, Inc., Rockville, MD, © 1986.]

Azimuthal Focus

Sound pulses suffer divergence in three dimensions, not just two. As a result, the pulse width increases in the third dimension perpendicular to the anatomic scanplane displayed onscreen. Increasing thickness of the anatomic scanplane may not obviously impact on the visual quality of the image, but directly influences another application of ultrasound imaging, that of guidance of invasive procedures. An umbilical vein and a venipuncture needle may both be seen onscreen but not in fact be perfectly **coplanar** if the anatomic slice thickness is increased. Most transducers manufacture the crystals in a curved shape to produce a minimum slice thickness at a permanent predetermined depth, use electronic focusing to optimize visual clarity in the image, and use different frequency transducers to optimize resolution in different applications (Fig. 1-12).

REVERBERATION ARTIFACT

Returning echoes will encounter surfaces on the way back to the transducer and produce new echoes at those surfaces. These subechoes will then encounter surfaces deeper and so on, essentially reverberating within tissue compartments. The machine cannot distinguish the weaker relatives of primary echoes from real

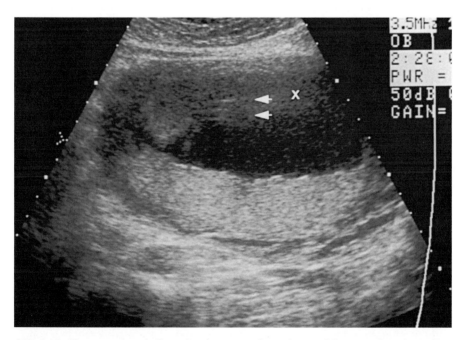

FIG. 1-13. The *arrows* here indicate the phantom surfaces that result from reverberation artifact, while the *x* indicates the general haze that also may result from reverberations in the heavy patient.

echoes until the period of programmed listening ends. These weak reverberated echoes will produce one of two visual phenomena. One such phenomenon is phantom surfaces deeper to the real tissues that demonstrate a regular repeat sequence but are weaker with each repeat. The other is the general overlay of low-grade echoes over the entire field of view (commonly seen with heavy patients) that interpose thick layers of tissue between the transducer and the anatomy of interest (Fig. 1-13).

SAFETY AND BIOHAZARD OF ULTRASOUND

The growing awareness over the past century that medical devices or interventions that appear harmless at first may hold hidden or delayed biohazards for the provider or the patient continues to motivate research into potential biohazards of ultrasound. Despite over 40 years of medical application of ultrasound no reproducible biohazard to the human fetus from imaging ultrasound has been reported.

The primary sources of biohazard from ultrasound are **heat** and **cavitation.** As we know, the kinetic energy of ultrasound is gradually transferred to the tissue as heat. **Documented thermal injury from imaging systems has not been reported.** Imaging systems use pulse echo designs that reduce actual energy exposure to 0.1% of any exposure time interval. Imaging systems use pulse power of extremely low order (less than 100 milliwatts per cm^2 at the transducer surface). **Cavitation** refers to a potentially explosive change in volume of microscopic bubbles of gas trapped within the tertiary structure of tissue proteins when exposed to pulses of high and low pressure as in the path of an ultrasound beam. Such explosive volume changes have the potential of damaging the proteins that might be critical to the organism. **Documented cavitational injury from imaging systems has not been reported.**

However, despite the fact that documented injury from imaging systems has not been reported, it remains prudent to limit ultrasound exposure to that which is medically necessary and informative. Lack of reported injury does not, in fact, prove safety conclusively. Exposure in the context of training should satisfy a clinical need as well. Exposure for nonmedical purposes is best minimized.

IMAGE DEVELOPMENT

The freehand nature of the linear or curvilinear array realtime transducer is both a blessing and a burden for the sonographer or sonologist. The ease of movement and the instant update of the visual information displayed on the screen provides insight into a large variety of biophysical information relevant to fetal well-being. However, the burden is on the examiner to move the transducer in methodical and productive ways. The most common error made early in a sonographic career is to move the transducer too **rapidly and randomly** hoping something familiar will be seen.

A logical plan, producing complete and methodical visualization of the uterine contents, the fetus, and the adnexae is required. Placement of the transducer in the vertical suprapubic midline, movement toward the fundus with a sweeping movement, then placement in the transverse suprapubic midline and sliding toward the fundus is a standard approach that will provide a complete viewing of the uterine contents. During this initial survey, the transducer should be aligned with the sagittal or the transverse planes of the mother. Later, the scanplane will be aligned with the fetus.

Format

Adoption and disciplined use of a consistent format for the viewed image on-screen will dramatically simplify visual interpretation of ultrasound images and minimize misinterpretation. The standard format for sagittal scanplane images is to display the caudal anatomy including maternal bladder and cervix to the right of the onscreen image, and the uterine fundus to the left (Fig. 1-14). This is anal-

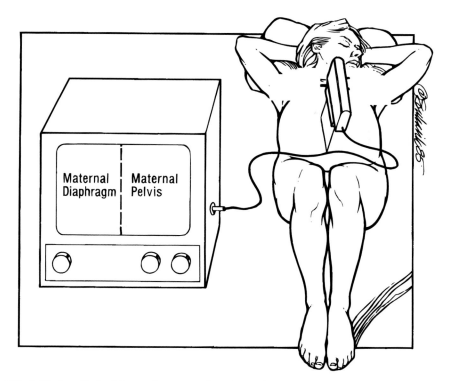

FIG. 1-14. Longitudinal format by convention places the maternal pelvis to the right of the viewscreen and the uterine fundus to the left. [Source: Reprinted from *Practical Obstetrical Ultrasound* (p. 23) by J. W. Seeds and R. C. Cefalo, Aspen Publishers, Inc., Rockville, MD, © 1986.]

ogous to standing at the right side of the bed looking at a sagittal section of maternal or intrauterine anatomy. This way, if the fetal vertex is to the right, you may always conclude the fetus is in a cephalic presentation, and, if the breech is to the right, you may conclude a breech presentation. Failure to adopt a standard format results in chaos. You must reorient yourself every time you pick up the transducer, and you must reorient every movement of the transducer to follow the new format. The standard format for transverse imaging is to display the patient's right to the left of the onscreen image, and her left, to the right (Fig. 1-15). This is analogous to standing at the foot of the bed looking at a transverse section of anatomy.

Transducer Movement

There are three basic transducer movements that include slide, angle, and rotation Fig. 1-16A,B,C). Often movements are complex combinations of these

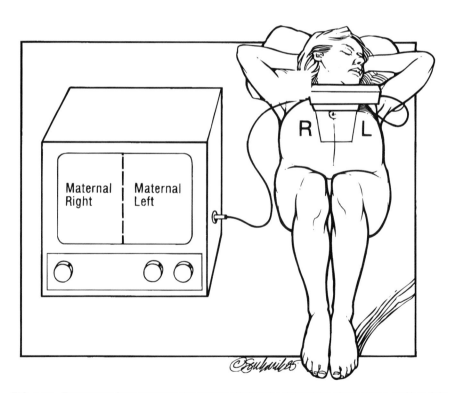

FIG. 1-15. Transverse format places the maternal left to the right of the viewscreen, and her right to the left. It is as if the viewer is at the foot of the bed looking at a transverse section of anatomy. [Source: Reprinted from *Practical Obstetrical Ultrasound* (p. 22) by J. W. Seeds and R. C. Cefalo, Aspen Publishers, Inc., Rockville, MD, © 1986.]

A

B

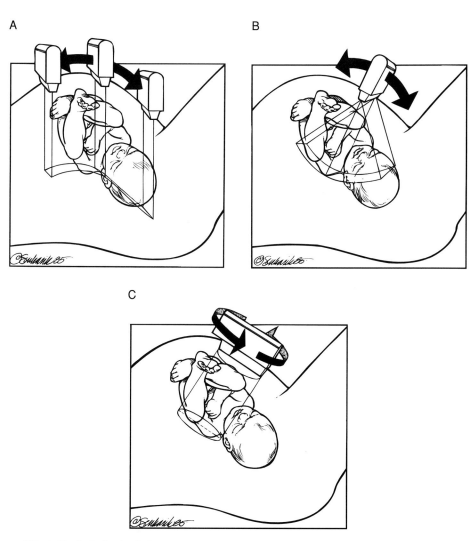

C

FIG. 1-16. A: A simple sliding movement of the freehand transducer will allow the examination of the contents of the uterus from a vertical viewpoint. **B:** Changing the angle of entry from a single contact point, allows manipulation of the scanplanes of fetal anatomy. **C:** Rotation of the transducer allows proper alignment of the scanplane with the anatomy of interest. [Source: Reprinted from *Practical Obstetrical Ultrasound* (p. 24–26) by J. W. Seeds and R. C. Cefalo, Aspen Publishers, Inc., Rockville, MD, © 1986.]

three, but, occasionally, discrete use of each is needed. Beginning in the suprapubic midline, while watching the anatomy unfold onscreen, sliding the transducer cephalad, and angling side to side, the entire uterine contents may be seen. Movement should not exceed the operator's ability to understand the anatomy. Excessively rapid transducer movement is the most common error made.

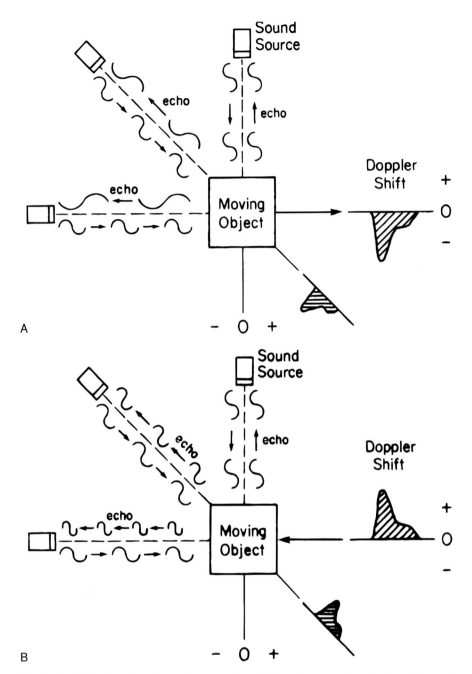

FIG. 1-17. A: The Doppler effect in the case of an object moving away from the transducer is to decrease the frequency or produce a negative Doppler shift. If the object is moving in a direction at a right angle to the direction of sound propagation, no Doppler shift is produced. If the object is moving directly away from the transducer **(zero angle)**, a maximal shift is produced. **B:** A positive Doppler shift is seen if the object is moving toward the transducer. [Source: Reprinted from *Congenital Malformations: Antenatal Diagnosis, Perinatal Management, and Counseling* (p. 38) by J. W. Seeds and R. G. Azizkhan, Aspen Publishers, Inc., Rockville, MD, © 1990.]

Once an adequate survey of uterine and intrauterine anatomy is completed, attention is focused on fetal anatomy and orientation may change. Scanplanes are best now chosen to relate to fetal axis, not maternal. Anatomic interpretation is greatly facilitated by proper longitudinal or transverse alignment of scanplane with fetal anatomy. Scanplanes oblique to fetal anatomy greatly complicate interpretation and are completely unnecessary.

Difficult and awkward at first, the operator quickly learns to move the transducer deliberately and slowly from one anatomic area to another using a knowledge of normal anatomy. Moving from the fetal head to the chest to the abdomen to the extremities in a logical and methodical fashion facilitates thoroughness. Future chapters will carefully examine specific components of the obstetric ultrasound examination such as normal fetal anatomy, fetal biometry, and selected malformations.

DOPPLER

The past decade has seen a remarkable interest in the use of Doppler ultrasound in obstetrics. Whether Doppler techniques prove to be of widespread benefit in obstetrics, Doppler ultrasound does provide additional diagnostic information into many specific clinical conditions, and a basic understanding of the principles of Doppler ultrasound is recommended.

A sound pulse generated from or reflected from a moving object demonstrates the **Doppler effect,** which is a change in the frequency. If the object is moving toward the receiver, the frequency increases and is called a **positive Doppler shift** (Fig. 1-17A,B). If the object is moving away from the receiver, the frequency is decreased, called a **negative Doppler shift**. The shift in frequency is proportional to the velocity of movement and is maximal if the direction of movement is exactly parallel to the direction of propagation of the sound pulses or toward the transducer, also called **zero angle.** If the direction of movement is 90 degrees to the direction of propagation of the primary sound pulse, there is no change in frequency.

TYPES OF DOPPLER SYSTEMS

Continuous Wave Doppler

Fetal monitors, office Dopplers, and some available Doppler umbilical artery devices generate ultrasound energy continuously at low amplitude and receive and analyze echoes continuously. Any Doppler shift anywhere along the soundpath is recorded, and, therefore, extraneous movement may confuse the information provided. Incorporation of continuous wave Doppler into imaging systems is not possible, because continuous sound generation would interfere with the imaging sound pulses. Therefore, there are severe limitations on the clinical usefulness of continuous systems. The operator cannot know precisely which vessel is being **interrogated,** or the **angle of insonation,** or where along the path of the vessel interrogation is taking place. Without the angle of insonation, relative assessment of systolic and diastolic velocities in the case of pulsatile arterial waveforms are possible, but the precise estimation of velocity is not possible.

Duplex Doppler

The analysis of Doppler shift of reflected echoes in a pulse-echo system allows incorporation into imaging systems, producing a Duplex Doppler system (Fig. 1-8). Such systems allow visualization of the vessel being interrogated, estimation of the angle of insonation, and, therefore, estimation of the actual velocity of movement. Such systems are substantially more expensive than continuous wave systems, but they provide significantly more information.

Color Flow Mapping

If echoes within a two-dimensional image are analyzed for Doppler shift in addition to geometric image information used to construct an image, and, if a color is assigned to those echoes in which a Doppler shift is detected and red is as-

PULSE DOPPLER DUPLEX

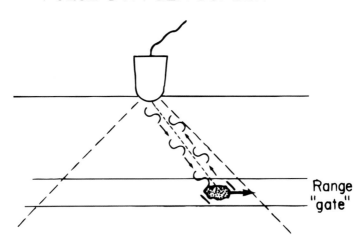

FIG. 1-18. Pulse Doppler incorporates the Doppler system into an imaging transducer and allows the user to visualize the blood vessel being interrogated and measure the angle of interrogation. The user may program the machine to analyze only echoes from a given depth, or "range gate" the process. [Source: Reprinted from *Congenital Malformations: Antenatal Diagnosis, Perinatal Management, and Counseling* (p. 39) by J. W. Seeds and R. G. Azizkhan, Aspen Publishers, Inc., Rockville, MD, © 1990.]

signed to positive Doppler shifts and blue to negative Doppler shifts, and, if the shade of color is related to the degree of shift, then the blood flowing within a realtime image might be colored red or blue and demonstrate in a visually dynamic fashion the cardiodynamic characteristics of a living system. This is the remarkable basis for color flow mapping. Color Doppler may demonstrate dynamic anatomic relationships such as blood flow within an abnormal fetal heart or locate a fetal blood vessel otherwise difficult or impossible to visually detect, either to facilitate pulse Doppler interrogation or blood sampling. The clinically necessary applications of color Doppler are limited.

COMMON TERMS

Sonographer   Non-M.D. technician or technologist trained and skilled in the performance of ultrasound examinations. It is recommended that these individuals undertake a specific course of instruction and pass the examinations and requirements to achieve certification as a Registered Diagnostic Medical Sonographer (RDMS). Such certification is required for practice in some localities.

Sonologist   M.D. or equivalent individual trained and skilled in the performance of ultrasound examinations. Although no national examination for competence is yet offered, evidence of training and experience, such as certification by an American Board that includes ultrasound skills, such as the American Board of Radiology or the American Board of Obstetrics and Gynecology, is encouraged.

Transducer   Device that converts electronic information into ultrasound pulses. These may be **linear array, curvilinear array, mechanical sector, endovaginal,** or **duplex Doppler.**

Coupling media   Any medium that couples the surface of the transducer to the skin surface of the patient by excluding the thin layer of air that would remain between a dry transducer and dry skin.

Acoustical Window   A fluid-filled organ such as bladder or ovarian cyst that, by virtue of the homogeneity of its contents, generates no echoes and thereby preserves maximum ultrasound intensity deeper into the patient to **enhance** the visualization of deep pelvic anatomy.

Acoustical Shadowing   The blocking of visualization of anatomy deep to bone or other anatomic structure that either reflects or blocks the sonographic pulses.

Reverberation Artifact   False images produced by stray echoes that reverberate within maternal or fetal tissue compartments, with the escape of a portion of the energy with each reverberation, producing the false image of a progressively deeper surface of progressively diminishing intensity. Typically, this phenomenon produces a generalized snowy overlay in heavy patients.

Anechoic   Lacking echoes, generally depicted as black. Related terms include echopenic, echoespared, echopoor.

Static   Lacking movement.

Realtime   The depiction of movement onscreen in realtime.

Grayscale   The adjustment of intensity of each pixel of the display to be proportional to the intensity of the echo analogous to that pixel.

Grayscale Emphasis Curve   The arbitrary modification of the grayscale proportionality to enhance visual clarity or visual perception.

Pulse Doppler   The analysis of Doppler shift of echoes generated from moving objects within a pulse-echo system.

Duplex Doppler   The incorporation of a pulse Doppler system within an imaging system.

Range Gate   The ability of a system to analyze Doppler shift of echoes from a specified depth along the sound propagation path.

2

Endovaginal Ultrasound

The ability to approximate pelvic structures by the use of endovaginal ultrasound probes allows the use of higher frequency transducers. The image quality is enhanced secondary to improved resolution, and, hence, a more definitive characterization of tissue texture is possible.

EQUIPMENT

A variety of scanning probes are available with varying angulation of the sector scanning beam and width of the scanning sector. Rotational probes are also available but are rarely used in clinical gynecologic scanning in the USA.

The use of transducers that emit the sector beam without angulation are designated "end-fire" transducers. These types of transducers were the first endovaginal probes in the United States and remain popular because of the ease in determining the scanning direction. Other probes emit the scanning sector area at an angle. The angulation varies with the specific manufacturer. Use of these probes may allow thorough scanning with less movement of the entire transducer. Use of any of these probes allows a natural interface between the bimanual pelvic exam and endovaginal sonography.

Because the probe is utilized within the vagina, a sheath (condom or glove) must be placed over the transducer for each patient. A coupling medium is placed within the sheath to cover the scanning tip and, in appropriate patients, a sterile lubricant is placed over the tip of the sheathed transducer to facilitate insertion. It should be noted that, if concern regarding the lubricant exists, (infertility patients for example) water or olive oil may be used. Sonographers and sonologists should carefully glove for endovaginal scanning in the same manner that is utilized for bimanual pelvic examination. Strict adherence to published guidelines for bloodborne pathogens is imperative with endovaginal scanning.

Between patients the transducer should be thoroughly cleaned by rinsing and wiping any residue from the transducer and then soaked in an appropriate cleaning solution such as activated glutaraldehyde (Cidex, Metricide) or glutaraldehyde-phenate (Sporicidin) for at least 20 minutes at room temperature. These solutions should not be stored above eye level for staff safety. In addition, the solution should be evaluated for appropriate potency each day and not used after 14 days of activation.

Jimenez and Duff noted less contamination of the transducer when a surgical glove was used to sheathe the transducer when compared with a condom. In their study of 240 patients undergoing endovaginal ultrasound scanning, either technique resulted in some transducer contamination. Perforation rates were 3.1% for gloves and 6.9% with condoms. One case (0.78%) of post-procedure transducer contamination was noted utilizing a surgical glove as a sheath versus 8 (7.8%) when a condom was used. Therefore, even when appropriate sheathing is utilized, solution sterilization between patients is necessary.

The portion of the transducer that is sheathed should be totally immersed in the solution. The handle and cable of the transducer should not be immersed in the cleansing solution.

SCANNING TECHNIQUE AND IMAGE FORMATTING

The endovaginal scanning session should begin with careful attention to the history and physical findings. A bimanual pelvic examination will assist in guiding the examination to assess the specific anatomy in question. Scanning should begin at the introitus with visualization of the vagina, bladder, and cervix as the transducer is inserted. In some patients, anxiety may be lessened if the patient is allowed to accomplish initial insertion of the transducer.

Gradually, the transducer is advanced into a fornix for assessment of pelvic anatomy. During manipulation of the pelvic viscera with the transducer, the normal sliding of organs and structures over peritoneal surfaces should be noted. If organs are fixed and do not readily slide, one must be concerned about adhesive processes precluding this movement.

With these transducers, one can achieve sagittal, oblique, and coronal scanning planes throughout the pelvis. Two primary transducer orientations are initially utilized with the scanning probe, a sagittal orientation with the reference guide superior; and a coronal orientation with the reference guide rotated 90 degrees counterclockwise to the patient's right. Obviously, intermediate scanning planes can also be achieved.

Utilizing this scanning approach, the image format during sagittal scanning will depict the ventral anatomy to the left side of the image (as it is viewed by the sonographer/sonologist) and dorsal anatomy to the right. In the coronal (transverse) plane, the patient's right pelvic anatomy will be depicted on the left of the image analogous to looking at the patient from the foot of the table or similar to the orientation of a bimanual pelvic examination (Fig. 2-1).

Once the viscera of interest is in the scanning field, the transducer can be oriented in such a manner to maximize the image quality. Appropriate image formatting (orienting the anatomy in the standard manner) is important in order to allow meaningful orientation of the anatomy and depiction of situs.

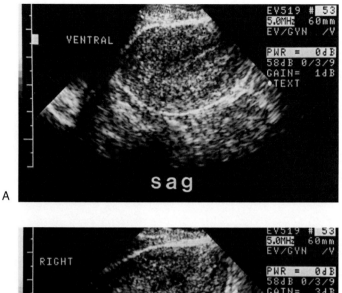

FIG. 2-1. In the sagittal plane **(A)** ventral anatomy is displayed to the viewer's left and dorsal to the right. In the coronal plane **(B)** the patient's right anatomy is displayed to the viewer's left and vice versa.

Equally important in gynecologic scanning is the image orientation of the particular viscera being studied in order to allow appropriate description of the anatomy that exists. Frequent use of labeling should be used to clarify anatomy and orientation. In other words, it is important to utilize patient-specific as well as organ-specific scanning planes.

In order to allow easier scanning with less transducer manipulation, many endovaginal probes have been constructed that have an angled sector field of view as noted above. The amount of angulation and the width of the sector image vary. Utilizing these endovaginal probes allows scanning of the pelvis with less movement of the transducer handle (Figs. 2-2,2-3,2-4).

A word of caution is necessary at this point. When manipulating the transducer, care must be taken not to create confusion regarding anatomic orientation. For example, in the sagittal plane, if the handle of the probe is tilted down to im-

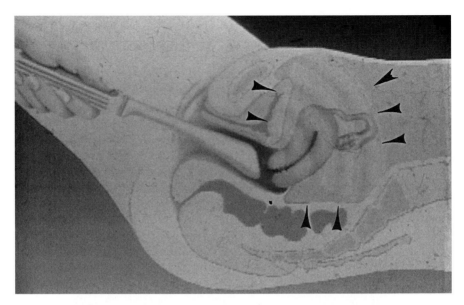

FIG. 2-2. Orientation of the intravaginal transducer in the mid-sagittal plane. Note the angulation of the imaging plane and the limits of the scan image (arrowheads). Realize that the image display will have the narrowest portion of the field of view at either the top or bottom of the monitor screen. (Courtesy of Acuson, Mountain View, CA.)

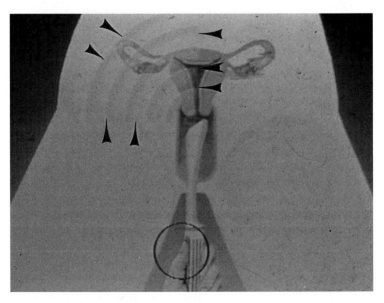

FIG. 2-3. Orientation of the intravaginal transducer in a coronal plane scanning the right adnexal area. The transducer was rotated in a counterclockwise 90-degree rotation. Notice the limits of the field of view (arrowheads). (Courtesy of Acuson, Mountain View, CA.)

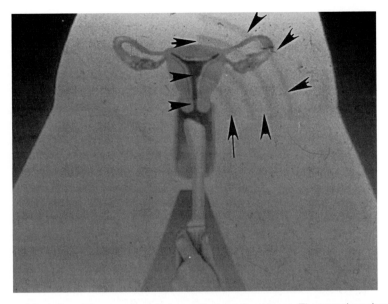

FIG. 2-4. Orientation of the transducer to image the left adnexal area. The transducer has been rotated 90 degrees clockwise from the mid-sagittal plane. This orientation results in a reversed orientation of right and left on the image unless the image direction orientation is changed. Notice the limits of the field of view *(arrowheads)*. (Courtesy of Acuson, Mountain View, CA.)

age more of the ventral anatomy, these structures will appear more inferiorly on the monitor. In addition, whereas the initial sagittal plane and right adnexa are insonated as mentioned above, some would recommend rotating the transducer 90 degrees clockwise from the sagittal plane (or the patient's left) to view the left adnexa. If this is done without changing the image direction display, the image format observed will be reversed regarding the right and left sides of the patient. To overcome this confusion the image may be reversed utilizing the "image direction" keyboard function. One must remember to reset the image direction to the standard format to avoid confusion and erroneous designation of organ orientation or situs in subsequent scans. Scanning of a retroverted uterus by rotating the probe 180 degrees and not altering the image direction may result in the same type of error. To avoid these pitfalls, the sonographer/sonologist should always re-evaluate the orientation of the image and the organ being studied.

The basic scanning procedure varies with individual preference of the sonographer/sonologist. A small amount of urine will assist in locating the anterior fornix of the vagina as the endovaginal probe is inserted through the introitus. Scanning of the pelvis should begin at the introitus and proceed cephalad. The cervix will be the initial structure visualized in most instances (Fig. 2-5).

The uterine fundus should then be located and an assessment of the position of the fundus in relationship to the cervix and pelvis is documented (i.e., retroversion, mid-position, anteversion) (Figs. 2-6, 2-7). The myometrium and en-

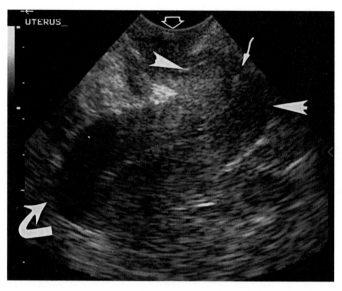

FIG. 2-5. Insertion of the vaginal transducer allows visualization of the vagina *(open arrow),* cervix *(large arrowheads),* external cervical os *(small arrow),* and fundus *(curved arrow).* Note the endometrial echo appearing as a "stripe" within the myometrium of this anteverted uterus.

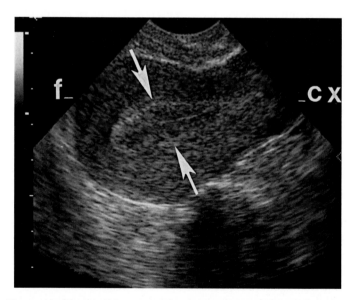

FIG. 2-6. Transvaginal image of an anteverted uterus demonstrating the fundus *(f)* and cervix *(cx).* The large arrows denote a prominent endometrium compatible with the secretory phase.

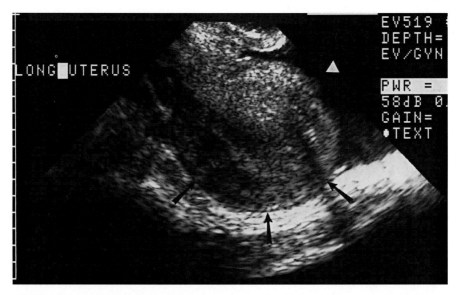

FIG. 2-7. Transvaginal image of a retroverted uterus. The fundus *(black arrows)* is oriented toward the cul-de-sac *(white arrowhead)*.

dometrium can then be evaluated. The contour of the uterus, shape of the fundus, presence of leiomyomata, thickness of the endometrium, and the texture of the endometrium are sequentially evaluated in the sagittal and coronal planes. Measurements of uterine size and endometrial thickness are then performed if desired.

The probe is then slowly manipulated into the right vaginal fornix. Slight rotation of the probe in the counterclockwise direction will facilitate visualization of the utero-ovarian relationship that exists. The underlying internal iliac vessels (hypogastric artery and vein) should be visible in the infero-lateral portion of the image. Occasionally, interposed bowel will obscure the ovary and gentle manipulation of the anterior abdominal wall by an abdominal hand (analogous to the bimanual examination) will allow the ovary to be visualized. If the ovary is still inapparent, orientation of the transducer in a coronal plane and sequentially scanning the adnexal area from ventral to dorsal will allow visualization of the ovary in the majority of cases (Fig. 2-8).

Two options exist to image the left adnexa. The transducer may be simply directed into this area with the reference guide oriented to the patient's right (i.e., unchanged) and the adnexal region scanned in the coronal plane. This method results in the standard image format with the patient's right located on the left side of the image.

In an effort to lessen transducer manipulation and, hence, patient discomfort, an alternative technique, especially suited for angled transducers involves returning to the mid-sagittal plane and then performing a clockwise rotation of the

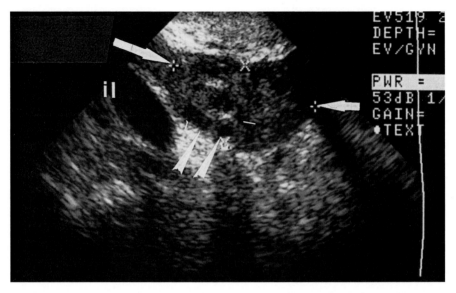

FIG. 2-8. The ovary is visualized in the adnexal region usually overlying the hypogastric (internal iliac) vessels *(il)*. This ovary is noted to be 2.1 × 3.9 cm by the calipers and the large white arrows. The ovarian stroma is normal and small follicles are seen *(arrowheads)*.

transducer 90 degrees from the sagittal plane (180 degrees from the coronal plane used for the right adnexa). The image direction function should be activated to display appropriate image formatting for appropriate documentation and later study.

Once the ovary is delineated, measurements in three planes will define the size and volume of the ovary. The presence or absence of ovarian masses is determined, and the masses, if any, are characterized. The evaluation of the ovary is most frequently performed in an organ-specific plane, (i.e., the maximum length, width, and thickness), and not a coronal or sagittal patient-specific plane. The number and size of preovulatory follicles are readily documented if desired.

Following completion of the endovaginal examination, the transducer is carefully removed to prevent any slippage of the covering sheath. As noted above, subclinical contamination of the transducer may occur. It is necessary, therefore, to appropriately sterilize the transducer between patients.

ADVANTAGES AND DISADVANTAGES OF ENDOVAGINAL SCANNING

As noted earlier, the endovaginal approach allows the scanning transducer tip to more closely approximate pelvic structures and, consequently, higher frequency transducers may be utilized with improved resolution and image quality. The disadvantage of endovaginal scanning relates to the decreased depth of field.

With this in mind, the need for transabdominal (transvesicle) scanning may exist for the evaluation of the pelvic mass that is distal to the field of view of the transducer being utilized. This need is particularly true to evaluate masses that are not in the true pelvis *per se*. One should not hesitate, therefore, to scan the patient utilizing both the endovaginal and the transabdominal approach in an effort to thoroughly visualize the entirety of the pelvis when necessary.

Another advantage of the endovaginal approach is that, by using the aspiration guide, directed aspiration procedures are possible. These procedures will be discussed in the chapter addressing complementary applications in gynecology.

In patients who cannot tolerate the insertion of the endovaginal probe, introital or transperineal imaging will allow imaging of the lower pelvic viscera. This technique is of particular benefit in prepubertal patients, some geriatric patients, and as an initial evaluation for possible placenta previa. This technique also requires appropriate sheathing of the transducer and bloodborne precautions by all staff involved.

If difficulty or discomfort is encountered while inserting the transducer, the patient may prefer to insert the probe. In many institutions this approach is routinely utilized in an effort to allow the patient to have more control of the procedure and thereby enhance patient cooperation. Because this type of ultrasound procedure is in reality a pelvic examination, regardless of gender, sonographers and sonologists should be encouraged to have an appropriate chaperon present during the examination.

SUMMARY

Endovaginal scanning has enhanced both the diagnostic accuracy and therapeutic potential of realtime ultrasound in the gynecologic patient. The natural interface between the bimanual pelvic examination and ultrasound has further established ultrasonography as an extension and enhancement of the pelvic examination.

Although the cost of endovaginal equipment is substantial, comprehensive assessment of the gynecologic patient by ultrasound requires this capability. When new equipment is sought, it is highly desirable to consider the feasibility of endovaginal capability.

FURTHER READING

Jimenez R, Duff P. Sheathing of the Endovaginal Ultrasound Probe: Is It Adequate? *J Infect Dis Obstet Gynecol* 1993;1:37–9.

3

A Road Map to the Screening Obstetric Sonogram

For the beginning sonographer, it can be overwhelming to think that you must be able to identify all abnormalities of fetal development. It is perhaps easier to learn to identify normal anatomy first, and then everything else is abnormal. Further definition, then, will depend on referring the patient to a tertiary level sonography center with whom you have a close relationship. After all, for most sonographers in practice, the goal is to provide screening studies and not diagnostic evaluations. It is critical for sonographers to understand the limits of their expertise and to be willing to ask for liberal consultation with others. It is perfectly acceptable to refer a patient for consultation when your screening study suggests an abnormality only to have the consultant consider the study normal; it is not acceptable for management of a pregnancy to change on the basis of an inexperienced sonographer's uncertain diagnosis.

Having emphasized liberal consultation in the case of unclear finding, the remainder of the chapter will deal with normal anatomy and which scanplanes to obtain when performing a screening ultrasound study of the second or third trimester fetus.

NORMAL ANATOMY

The period of organogenesis lasts until about 14 postmenstrual weeks. After that, organs are maturing and growing, but the intrinsic anatomy is present. Even so, the sonographic appearance of normally developed structures may change during pregnancy.

Ultrasound views of neural anatomy will change throughout gestation as different degrees of myelination occur, and the echodensity of brain will increase as pregnancy progresses. Similarly, the bowel will become more prominent as pregnancy progresses because meconium does not reach the cecum until about half way through pregnancy. Increased right ventricular pressure, as may occur with placental insufficiency, may cause an increase in the size of the right atrium due to the increased right heart pressure, resulting in asymmetry of an otherwise normal heart.

It is important to recall that screening sonography of the second and third trimester features should include a detailed overview of fetal anatomy, as outlined by both the American Institute for Ultrasound in Medicine (AIUM) and American College of Obstetrics and Gynecology (ACOG) (see also Chapter 4).

CENTRAL NERVOUS SYSTEM

Central nervous system (CNS) abnormalities are among the most common and most serious malformations that affect the fetus. Consequently, screening sonography should assess intracranial anatomy. Filly and others showed that the minimum assessment of intracranial anatomy that would exclude over 90% of fetal intracranial abnormalities include demonstration of a normal **cavum septum pellucidum,** normal **posterior horns of lateral ventricles** and **normal posterior fossa** (Figs. 3-1–3-3). The cavum septum pellucidum appears as an echolucent, narrow widening in the midline echo on the biparietal diameter (BPD) view, anterior to the thalamus and about one third of the way between the frontal bone and the thalamus. Absence of the cavum is a marker for agenesis of the corpus callosum. By rotating the transducer slightly toward the occiput from the BPD view, the posterior fossa view is obtained. The posterior fossa contains the cerebellar hemispheres, cisterna magna, and the nuchal skin fold. The most common

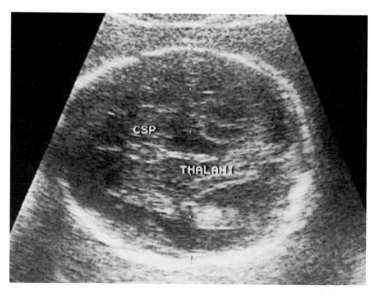

FIG. 3-1. The scan plane used to measure the BPD should include the cavum septum pellucidum, thalami, and should exclude the posterior horns of the lateral ventricles and posterior fossa. CSP, cavum septum pellucidum.

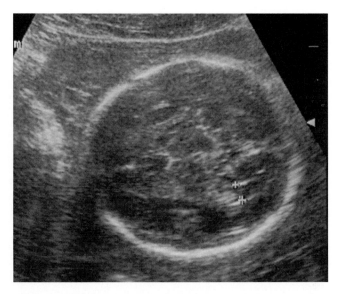

FIG. 3-2. By rotating the transducer slightly posteriorly from the BPD view, the posterior tip of the choroid plexus should be seen, outlined by an anechoic rounded structure, which is the posterior horn of the lateral ventricle.

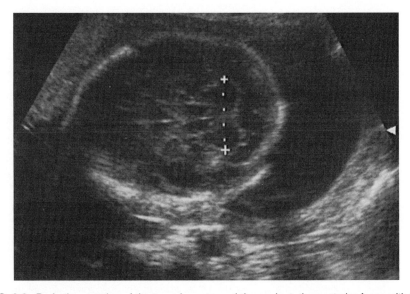

FIG. 3-3. By further rotation of the transducer toward the occiput, the posterior fossa with the paired cerebellar hemispheres and hypoechoic cisterna magna should be seen.

disorder that distorts this view is open spina bifida, which causes contents of the posterior fossa to be pulled through the foramen magnum into the upper neck, obliterating the cisterna magna and compressing the cerebellar hemispheres (banana sign) (Fig. 3-4). Other CNS malformations that can distort this view include Dandy-Walker cyst with an enlarged cisterna magna, widely separated cerebellar hemispheres, and a defect in the vermis of the cerebellum (Fig. 3-5). In addition, a hypoplastic cerebellum may be associated with some chromosomal abnormalities (Fig. 3-6). Midway between the two scanplanes, there should be clear definition of the posterior horn of the lateral ventricles. Since this is the lowest pressure area of the lateral ventricular system, disorders that cause lateral ventriculomegaly will cause enlargement of this area first and worst. The posterior horn should measure less than or equal to 10 mm in fetuses at 20 weeks or less.

In addition to these three views, the sonographer should assess that the midline is symmetric and that the shape of the fetal head is normal (Figs. 3-7–3-9).

The fetal spine should be examined both longitudinally and transversely throughout its length. It is vital to remember that the cervical spine widens to sup-

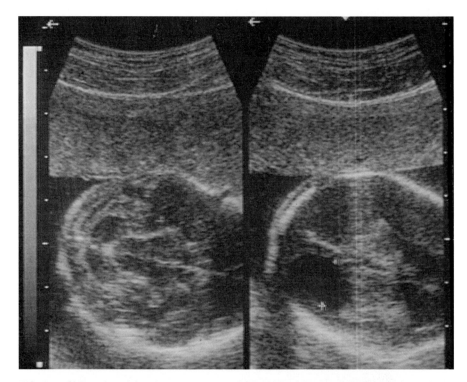

FIG. 3-4. Obliteration of the cisterna magna and flattening of the cerebellar hemispheres in the Arnold-Chiari II malformation that accompanies most cases of fetal open spina bifida will produce the so-called banana sign, seen on the left side of this figure. The right side shows the accompanying lateral ventriculomegaly also.

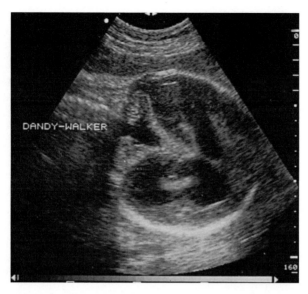

FIG. 3-5. The ultrasound findings of a Dandy-Walker malformation include cystic dilation of the cisterna magna, splaying of the cerebellar hemispheres, and a defect in the vermis of the cerebellum.

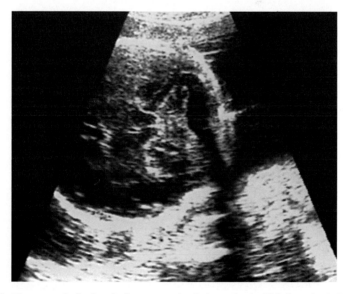

FIG. 3-6. These cerebellar hemispheres are clearly hypoplastic. This fetus had trisomy 18.

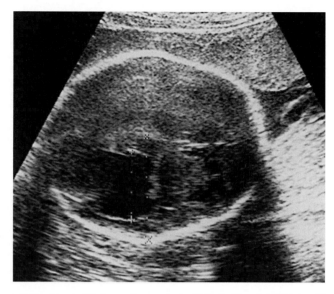

FIG. 3-7. The posterior horn in this image is massively dilated with only a thin rim of brain tissue at the periphery. The lack of detail in the leading hemisphere is a common problem, due to reverberation artifact.

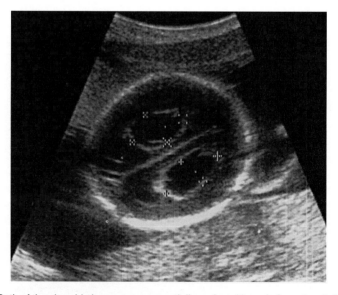

FIG. 3-8. Both of the choroid plexuses are essentially replaced by echolucent cysts in this fetus with trisomy 18.

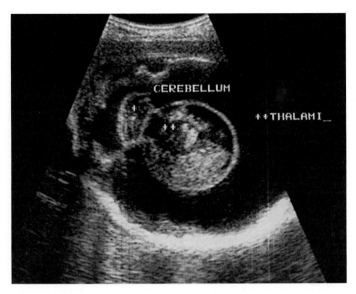

FIG. 3-9. This image shows the distorted midbrain and fluid-filled cranium without cerebral tissue but a relatively intact cerebellum in a fetus with hydranencephaly.

port the head, but that, below the level of the cervical spine, the echocenters of the spine should be roughly parallel in longitudinal view. A full description of the scanplanes used to diagnose open spina bifida is included in Chapter 9.

ABDOMEN

The **abdominal circumference** is measured in a scanplane perpendicular to the fetal spine, such that multiple rib cross sections are seen. The fetal stomach should be seen, as should the straight segment of the umbilical vein. By sliding the transducer caudally to the fetus, maintaining a perpendicular orientation, both kidneys should be visualized. Both kidneys should be routinely visualized after 18 weeks; it is not uncommon to see them clearly by transvaginal scanning as early as 12 weeks (Fig. 3-10). Fetal lobulations may be identified in the third trimester. Fluid collections within the kidney may be observed in the renal pelvis, with the normal anteroposterior dimension of the renal pelvis being 4 and 7 mm at under and over 30-weeks gestation, respectively. Late in the third trimester, individual calyces may normally be visualized. Further sliding of the transducer caudally should demonstrate the fetal bladder.

Returning to the abdominal circumference view, angle the transducer now cranially to the fetus. This should reveal a **four chamber view of the heart.** Many beginning sonographers are nervous about fetal heart assessment, but the principles are similar to evaluation of any other structure. Table 3-1 summarizes the criteria necessary to call a four chamber heart view "normal" (Fig. 3-11).

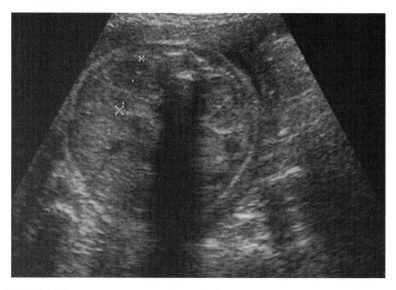

FIG. 3-10. The kidneys are seen as medium echodense, paired, round structures in this transverse view of the fetal abdomen. The one on the left has been measured in the anteroposterior (AP) diameter.

In this same plane, assess the lungs. They should be slightly more echodense than the liver and homogeneous (Fig. 3-12). The shapes of the lungs are slightly different, but the amount of lung tissue on the left and right sides should be approximately equal.

Four limbs should be identified. In addition, a careful survey of the placenta should allow a description of the position of the placenta and any gross pathology. If more than one fetus is present, document the presence of an intervening membrane.

TABLE 3-1. *Criteria for a normal four-chamber view of the fetal heart*

Heart should occupy $\frac{1}{3}$ to $\frac{1}{2}$ the chest.
Rate should be between 120 and 160 beats per minute.
The apex of the heart should point toward the fetal left side.
The foramen ovale should be seen in the left atrium.
The tricuspid valve should be displaced slightly on the ventricular septum relative to the mitral valve.
The atria should be symmetric.
The ventricles should be approximately equal in size and shape.
A line drawn from the dorsal echocenter of the spine to the sternum should cross the right ventricle.

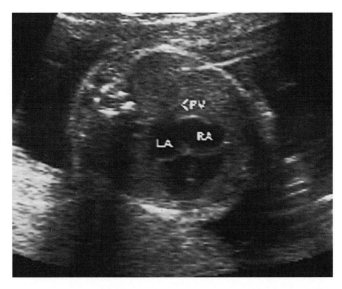

FIG. 3-11. A normal four-chambered view of the heart should have the features listed in Table 3-1. The lungs are seen surrounding the heart. LA, left atrium; RA, right atrium; PV, pulmonary vein.

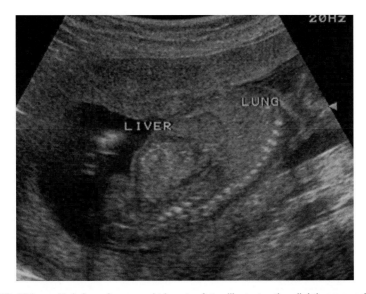

FIG. 3-12. This sagittal view of a second trimester fetus illustrates the slightly more echodense appearance of the lung compared to the liver.

SUMMARY

Careful inspection of the anatomic scanplanes is necessary. A mental or physical check list of pertinent anatomy, documenting not only what you have visualized, but also what has not been seen, may help in documenting the adequacy of the examination. Since the fetus rarely lies still long enough to allow a top-down approach to the anatomic survey, a flexible organization to the examination is necessary.

The interpreting physician is responsible for confirming that the appropriate anatomy has been examined, deciding whether the anatomy is normal, abnormal, or questionable, and then determining the next diagnostic step necessary, if any. Questionable findings should be confirmed by someone with further skills in the area of fetal sonography. Patients at significant risk for a fetal abnormality should have diagnostic scanning performed and not a screening sonogram.

FURTHER READING

Cardoza JD, Goldstein RB, Filly RA. Exclusion of fetal ventriculomegaly with a single measurement: the width of the lateral ventricular atrium. *Radiology* 1988;169:711–4.

Filly RA, Cardoza JD, Goldstein RB, Barkovich AJ. Detection of fetal central nervous system anomalies: a practical level of effort for a routine sonogram. *Radiology* 1989;172(2):403–8.

Reed KL, Anderson CF, Shenker L. Fetal Echocardiography. In: *An Atlas*. New York: Wiley-Liss. 1988;12.

4

Guidelines for Obstetric Ultrasound

Obstetric sonography is a medical examination for which a clear indication should be stated and for which the operators should be adequately trained and interested to consistently perform the procedure with high quality. Each sonographer is responsible for understanding the potential limits of sonography as both a diagnostic and screening test, as well as his or her own limitations as a sonographer. The operator must be willing to accept the responsibility of performing fetal sonography and be willing to refer patients if indicated.

This chapter will describe indications for ultrasound during pregnancy, the data available regarding the potential utility of universal or routine ultrasound, and published guidelines for the minimum content of a basic fetal ultrasound examination.

Indications for ultrasound during pregnancy vary according to where one practices medicine. Routine ultrasound, as many as three per pregnancy, is a standard part of prenatal care in some countries. In the United States, the routine use of ultrasound has not been embraced on a national level, although the individual practitioner may make an independent decision. The National Institutes of Health (NIH) Consensus Development Conference in 1984 resulted in a list of specific indications for obtaining prenatal sonography. These are listed in Table 4-1.

A call for a randomized study to address the potential utility of universal screening in the United States was included in the NIH Consensus Report. The results of such a study, the so-called RADIUS study (Routine Antenatal Diagnostic Imaging With Ultrasound) were reported in 1993. From an initial population of about 57,000 registrants for prenatal care in the study population, approximately 15,000 were eligible to participate. This highly selected group of women were at low risk for any poor maternal or poor fetal outcome. It comes as little surprise that the RADIUS study was unable to demonstrate an improvement in perinatal outcome in those women randomized to receive only "indicated" scans and those randomized to receive two routine scans. The average number of indicated scans in the control population was 0.6/woman. Several secondary out-

TABLE 4-1. Indications for prenatal sonography from the NIH
Consensus Development Conference, 1984

Uncertain last menstrual period
Evaluation of fetal growth
Vaginal bleeding of undetermined etiology in pregnancy
Determination of fetal presentation
Suspected multiple gestation
Adjunct to amniocentesis
Significant uterine size/clinical dates discrepancy
Pelvic mass
Suspected hydatidiform mole
Adjunct to cervical cerclage
Suspected ectopic pregnancy
Adjunct to special procedures (fetoscopy, cordocentesis, CVS, IVF)
Suspected fetal death
Suspected uterine abnormality
Intrauterine contraceptive device localization
Ovarian follicle development surveillance
Biophysical evaluation for fetal well-being
Observation of intrapartum events (version, second twin)
Manual removal of placenta
Suspected polyhydramnios or oligohydramnios
Suspected abruption
Adjunct to external cephalic version
Estimation of fetal weight
Abnormal serum alphafetoprotein
Follow-up observation of identified anomaly
Follow-up of placenta location for placenta previa
History of prior congenital anomaly
Serial evaluation of fetal growth in multiple gestation
Evaluation of fetal condition in late registrants for care

CVS, chorionic villus sampling; IVF, *in vitro* fertilization.

comes approached a significant level of improvement in the routinely scanned women but failed to meet statistical levels of improvement. Importantly, the detection rate of fetal defects was higher in those women scanned at tertiary medical centers compared with those scanned in private offices.

The practical answer for the individual obstetric care provider regarding the use of routine versus selected ultrasound must be drawn from scientific studies evaluated in the context of one's own practice. According to the American College of Obstetrics & Gynecology (ACOG), over 70% of American pregnancies undergo prenatal ultrasound. If a practice includes many women with high-risk factors for adverse maternal and fetal outcomes and the facilities and personnel to perform an appropriate level of ultrasound examination are reasonably available in the community, then routine sonography may make sense.

Reimbursement issues will also affect whether sonography can be considered a routine part of obstetric care or only done on selected patients.

Once an ultrasound has been requested, it is important to understand what information should be garnered from the study. The terminology that has evolved around obstetric ultrasound, such as "Level I" and "II" or "basic" versus "targeted", acknowledges that some patients need a more extensive level of sonography than others. This differentiation has formed a schism between the basic sonographer who may resent the imposition of responsibility for an anatomic survey when the clinical question is What is the gestational age? and the specialist sonographer who contends that "sneaking a peak" is an inadequate use of the technology. Cogent opinions on either side of this argument exist. For instance, Benacerraf questions whether there should be Level I or II deliveries or should all accoucheurs be able to perform all deliveries? On the surface, this is a reasonable question, but, in reality, anyone delivering babies needs to be able to perform basic obstetric maneuvers, treat obstetric emergencies such as relief of a shoulder dystocia, and also to recognize when a patient should be referred for a specialist evaluation and treatment. In addition, a physician is expected to know how to take a history and perform a screening cardiac examination, but it is considered not only acceptable but appropriate for a patient with abnormal heart sounds or cardiovascular symptoms to be referred to a cardiologist to help define and treat the problems.

In a similar vein, there are two paradigms that form useful constructs of obstetric ultrasound. The first is the use of ultrasound as a **screening test.** Screening tests, by World Health Organization definition, are those applied to patients at low risk for a common, significant, treatable problem and that are relatively inexpensive, safe, and accurate. If one looks at the indications for ultrasound that were listed in the NIH Consensus Report, history taking and lab tests are screening tests that may be the basis for recommending an ultrasound in order to resolve the issue for which the screening test was abnormal. The ultrasound, then, may be considered a **diagnostic test** if it is able to accurately resolve the question raised.

For instance, the NIH Consensus Report lists uncertain last menstrual period (LMP) as an indication for ultrasound. A basic ultrasound, performed at less than 24 weeks, for gestational age assessment and including an overview of fetal anatomy would be considered a diagnostic test for assignment of an accurate gestational age but only a screening test for birth defects. Abnormal findings on the screening ultrasound should prompt the sonographer either to do a more in depth examination or to refer the patient to a qualified specialist.

For instance, given a patient with a clinically dated pregnancy who has a borderline elevated maternal serum alphafetoprotein (MSAFP), a reasonable next step in her evaluation would be to do a screening ultrasound, looking for reassignment of gestational age or an unsuspected multiple gestation. If a singleton fetus with no date change is found on initial sonography, it is reasonable to refer the patient to a center where people skilled in diagnostic ultrasound can examine the fetus for stigmata of open neural tube defects (ONTD) and other open fetal birth defects. These two paradigms are illustrated in Table 4-2. An important feature of both approaches is that additional information beyond that which is asked of the test is available from ultrasound and that, even under the best of circumstances, no ultrasound can be 100% accurate.

In order to wisely select patients for targeted sonography, it is helpful to understand the causes of most birth defects. This will allow you to identify at the beginning of prenatal care those pregnancies most at risk for a fetal birth defect so that appropriate prenatal testing can be requested. Although not exhaustive, Table 4-3 describes the mechanisms for many of the more common fetal disorders and identifies maternal characteristics that may put her in a high-risk group for these disorders, prompting a referral for targeted sonography.

In an effort to define the minimum content of obstetric ultrasound, the American Institute of Ultrasound in Medicine (AIUM) and the American College of Obstetrics & Gynecology (ACOG) have published guidelines for obstetric ultrasound. Table 4-4 describes these guidelines. There are many similarities and some subtle differences among them. In order to be granted ultrasound privileges at some institutions, liability insurance coverage, or reimbursement for performed ultrasounds, it may be necessary for the clinician to document adherence to one or another of these guidelines. More importantly, these guidelines provide an excellent framework for quality patient care.

Although these guidelines seem exhaustive, in reality it only takes about 10 to 15 minutes to perform the basic scans once experience is gained and a routine established. Just as the method of performance of a complete physical examination had to be learned and patterns established, the fetal ultrasound can be mastered, with patience, compulsive attention to detail, and practice.

It is vital that a standard, but flexible, approach be adopted. For first-trimester pregnancies, a combination of both transabdominal and transvaginal sonography may be needed. If a transabdominal scan fails to answer the clinical question, most commonly to confirm the presence of an *in utero,* viable embryo, then transvaginal scanning will be necessary. Chapter 5 details the first trimester examination.

For the most part, a second- or third-trimester screening ultrasound is performed with an empty, nondistended bladder using transabdominal techniques. Use the highest frequency transducer that will permit visualization of the anatomy, usually a 5.0 megahertz transducer during the second trimester and a 3.5 megahertz transducer later or in a heavy woman, one with significant abdominal scarring, or in the presence of polyhydramnios.

By beginning the scan with an overview of the uterine contents, the sonographer can quickly assess many of the points on the guidelines and rapidly orient to the fetus. Align the transducer longitudinally in the midline over the maternal pubic symphysis. The image on the screen should be oriented such that the maternal bladder and symphysis are on the right side of the screen and the presenting part visualized (Fig. 4-1). If permanent documentation is done using still frame images, one taken with this initial transducer placement will document

TABLE 4-2. Paradigms of ultrasound as a screening test and as a diagnostic test for certain clinical questions

Indications for scan	Optimal screening sonography	
	Diagnostic for	Screening for
Late prenatal care	Number	Most structural
Size unequal to dates	Viability	abnormalities
Uncertain LMP	Gestational age	
Suspected multiple gestation		
	Optimal referred sonography	
	Diagnostic for	Screening for
Abnormal Screening Sonogram	Most structural	Aneuploidy
Elevated MSAFP unexplained by	abnormalities	Metabolic and functional
screening sonogram		disorders
Prior structural anomalies		
Polyhydramnios/oligohydramnios		

LMP, last menstrual period.

TABLE 4-3. Mechanisms and risk factors for common fetal conditions

Type of fetal condition	Mechanism	Clinical association
1. Aneuploidy	Abnormal meiosis, usually involving the egg; usually causes multiple anomalies.	Advanced maternal age Previous aneuploidy ≤3 prior miscarriages Ultrasound dysmorphology Abnormal maternal serum screening
2. Teratogenic	Disruption of normal embryologic events	Seizure disorder Alcohol abuse Use of accutane periconceptionally
3. Infectious	Fetal or placental infection with either disruption of normal embryologic events or disruption of established tissues	Documented syphilis during pregnancy Viral serology Fetal growth restriction
4. Metabolic	Probably related to teratogenic insult	Maternal diabetes
5. Genetic	Single gene disorders	Family history of prior affected individuals—usually requires direct questioning
6. Growth restriction	Placental dysfunction Nutritional deprivation	Maternal hypertension Smoking Size < dates
7. Multifactorial	Unknown; probably multiple mechanisms	Family history Elevated AFP

TABLE 4-4. American Institute of Ultrasound in Medicine and American College of Obstetrics & Gynecology guidelines for content of a basic ultrasound examination

	AIUM	ACOG
Equipment	Realtime scanner Appropriate frequency Lowest possible settings	Realtime scanner Appropriate frequency, Type transducer: lowest reasonable settings

Documentation	Permanent, labeled images of
	  biometry, anatomy written
	  report	

Level of
  sonography
	Limited sonography may be
	  performed in clinical
	  emergency or as follow-up to
	  complete examination.
		Limited exam reasonable under
		  certain circumstances to get
		  specific information or under
		  urgent conditions.
		Basic ultrasound is primarily
		  metric but should include fetal
		  and maternal anatomy.
		Comprehensive exam indicated
		  when high risk for
		  physiologically or anatomically
		  abnormal fetus.

First trimester	Location gestational sac
	Identify embryo
	Crown-rump length
	Confirmation fetal life
	Fetal number
	Uterine/adnexal anatomy
		Presence/absence of intrauterine
		  sac
		Identification embryo or fetus
		Crown-rump length
		Presence/absence of cardiac
		  motion
		Fetal number
		Uterine/adnexal structures

Second/third
  trimester
	Fetal life
	Fetal number
	Fetal presentation
	Assessment amniotic fluid
	  volume
	Placental location/appearance
	Estimation gestational age using
	  BPD, femur
	Assess interval growth with serial
	  scans
	Uterine, adnexal examination
	Anatomic survey: cerebral
	  ventricles, 4-champber heart,
	  spine, stomach, bladder,
	  umbilical cord, renal region
		Fetal life
		Fetal number
		Fetal presentation
		Assessment amniotic fluid
		  volume
		Placental location
		Assessment gestational age
		
		Maternal pelvic masses
		Anatomic survey: cerebral
		  ventricles, 4-chamber heart,
		  spine, stomach, bladder, cord
		  insertion, renal region

fetal position. A slow sweep from pelvis to uterine fundus, maintaining a longitudinal orientation of the transducer but angling from side-to-side will quickly demonstrate cardiac activity, fetal number, placental location, subjective assessment of amniotic fluid volume, and fetal presentation. Completing this sweep by sliding the transducer to image the adnexal areas will allow one to screen for ad-

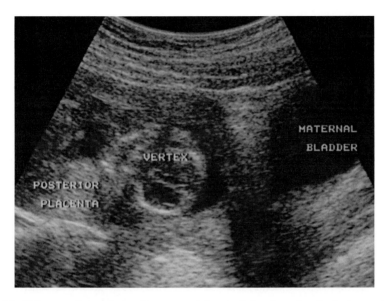

FIG. 4-1. This scan demonstrates the appropriate orientation for a longitudinal scan image, demonstrating the maternal bladder on the right, fetal vertex, and placenta posterior.

nexal pathology. Normal ovaries in late pregnancy may be difficult to image. Still-frame documentation of fetal cardiac activity is easily accomplished by freezing an M-mode image through the fetal heart (Fig. 4-2).

The two major remaining tasks, to determine gestational age and to perform an anatomic survey, are integrated processes because much of the important fetal anatomy will be visualized while developing the scanplanes for fetal measurement. In addition, some fetal anatomy can best be studied in certain fetal positions. If the fetal position is optimal for such a study while measurements are being performed, one should temporarily interrupt the biometry. Inevitably, if one chooses instead to complete the task of fetal measurement and then go back to document anatomy, the fetus will have moved to a suboptimal position. This approach will ultimately shorten the time necessary to complete the examination but demands that the sonographer maintain a flexible, yet thorough approach.

Most contemporary ultrasound units have standard charts for biometric data within the software of the machine. It is the sonographer's responsibility, however, to confirm that the charts used are compatible with his or her own population of patients and that the technique used by the author to generate those charts matches that used in clinical practice. This will eliminate some systematic errors.

Other possible sources of error include use of the wrong scanplane. For instance, the scanplane for the biparietal diameter (BPD) should show a symmetric, elliptical skull (Fig. 4-3). Midline brain structures should divide the cranial contents symmetrically. The midline falx at the level of the BPD should be discontinuous, interrupted about one quarter of the way posteriorly from the frontal bone by the cavum septum pellucidum. The thalami, posterior to the cavum sep-

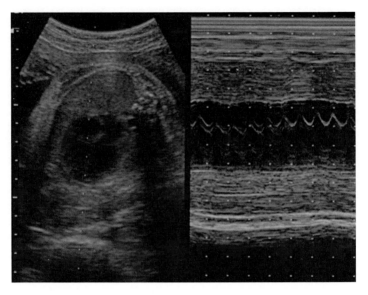

FIG. 4-2. Hard-copy documentation of fetal viability is possible using M-mode. On the left, a 2D image of the fetal heart is shown; the dotted line traversing the lung, right atrium, and ventricle and tricuspid valve is the M-line (motion line). On the right, the motion of the tricuspid valve under the M-line confirms fetal life.

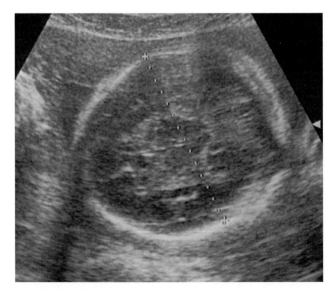

FIG. 4-3. The biparietal diameter (BPD) is the largest diameter, transverse to the fetal head, at the level of the thalami and cavum septum pellucidum.

tum pellucidum, also interrupt the falx. In the proper BPD scanplane, the posterior fossa is not visible. This is the same scanplane used to obtain the occipitofrontal diameter (OFD) and head circumference (HC). All measurements should be taken at least three times and averaged. If linear measurements differ by more than 1 mm they should be repeated, being cautious to obtain the proper scanplane and cursor placement. Circumference measurements should consistently be within 10% of each other.

The standard abdominal measurement is obtained in a plane perpendicular to the abdomen at the level of the liver, stomach, and the linear portion of the umbilical cord (Fig. 4-4). Kidneys, heart and lungs should not be seen. Cross-sections of multiple ribs should be seen, in distinction to an entire length of any one rib segment. The abdominal circumference (AC) is the only standard measurement that is predominantly soft tissue. Thus distortions that can cause the AC to be out of round are common sources of error. For instance, if the fetal legs are flexed against the abdomen or excessive pressure is applied over the abdomen with the transducer, the AC can be distorted. Therefore, the AC measurements are more variable from observer to observer and also with repeat measurements by the same observer, increasing the importance of triplicate measurements.

Long bones are among the easiest of fetal structures for which to confirm an appropriate scanplane but, due to the mobility of the limbs, can be the most difficult for the novice to obtain. Femur images may be obtained by sliding the transducer transversely down the length of the spine until the proximal head of the femur is identified. The transducer is then rotated around the femoral head image until the full length of the femur is obtained. The echodensity of the femur should be homogeneous. Both ends of the femur should be crisp, without blurring.

Scanplanes for some anatomic evaluations differ somewhat from those for biometric analysis. Obviously, the position and size of the stomach can be demonstrated while obtaining the AC. By imaging caudally from there, one easily obtains transverse images of both kidneys and bladder as well as the cord insertion, simply by angling and sliding the transducer (Fig. 4-5). From the AC plane, the four-chamber heart view can be obtained by angling the transducer cephalad to the fetus. Criteria for a normal four-chamber view are discussed fully in Chapter 11.

Intracranial anatomy is the most complex of the structures that must be assessed. As well, central nervous system (CNS) malformations are both common and serious. Filly and colleagues reported a retrospective review of sonograms of 112 fetuses throughout pregnancy with ultrasound-visible CNS malformations. In 95% there were abnormal measurements of the cisterna magna or atrial measurements of the posterior horns of the lateral ventricles, while the other 5% were grossly apparent. It seems reasonable, therefore, to include measurements of these structures in a screening study of intracranial anatomy.

The posterior horns of the lateral ventricles can be imaged by obtaining the BPD scanplane and then angling the transducer just slightly caudally toward the

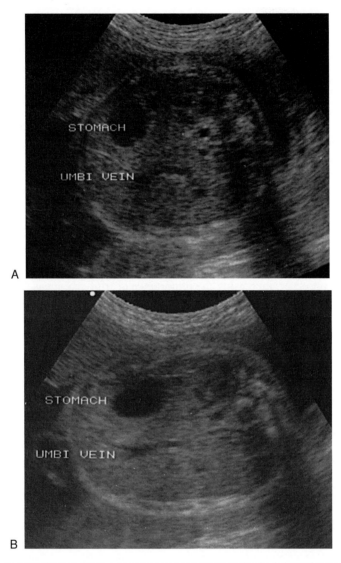

FIG. 4-4. Landmarks to confirm a proper scanplane for an abdominal circumference include the stomach, linear portion of the umbilical vein, and multiple cross-sections of ribs. Images **A** and **B** were obtained in the same fetus at the same scanplane. The distortion of the nice circular image of A was obtained by applying too much pressure with the transducer. If you get an elliptic abdominal circumference (AC), consider lightening up on your hand pressure.

cerebellum (Fig. 4-6). The choroid plexus fills the lateral ventricles, and the posterior horns are measured just beyond the posterior end of the choroid plexus. The measurement should be made perpendicular to the ventricle, not perpendicular to the midline. The posterior horn should not exceed 1.0 cm. Further angling of the transducer caudally will result in the image of the posterior fossa. The cis-

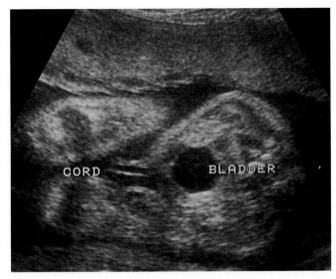

FIG. 4-5. A transverse view of the lower abdomen shows the bladder and umbilical cord insertion site. Both knees are visible just to the left of the cord insertion.

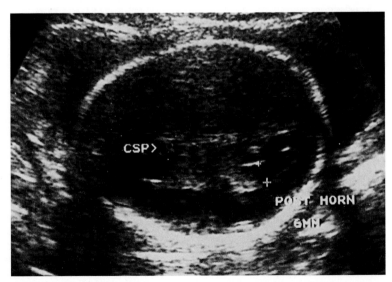

FIG. 4-6. The atrium of the posterior horn of the lateral ventricle dilates first and worst with fetal hydrocephalus. Its measurement, as shown here, should not exceed 1 cm throughout pregnancy.

terna magna is the echolucent space between the cerebellar hemispheres and the occipital bones (Fig. 4-7).

The neuraxis should be further examined by obtaining images of the fetal spine. There are three echodensities that represent ossification centers of each vertebra and lamina. In the presence of open spina bifida, the equilateral triangle formed by the two dorsal ossification centers and the ventral one is distorted due to splaying of the laminae of the vertebrae. Some spina bifida will have herniated meninges that may be seen as a cystic outpouching from the midline of the back, while others will be flat defects, suggested by either deviation of the spine itself or the abnormal positions of the ossification centers. The spinal views that should be obtained, therefore, include both transverse views through each vertebra imaging the three ossification centers and coronal views of the two dorsal ossification centers trying to image the splayed laminae.

If multiple fetuses are present, the examination should be completed on each one. Multiple gestations have increased rates of several perinatal complications, such as prematurity, abnormal fetal lie, growth abnormalities, and malformation. In general, these complications are more common with monozygotic twins, so a complete assessment of a multi-fetal gestation will include an assessment of probable zygosity, as well as gestational age assessment of anatomic survey. Depending on the point in early embryonic development that cleavage of the cell mass occurs, monozygotic twins can have completely separate membranes and placenta (diamniotic, dichorionic); a common placenta, but separate amnion (diamniotic, monochorionic); a common placenta and amnion (monoamniotic,

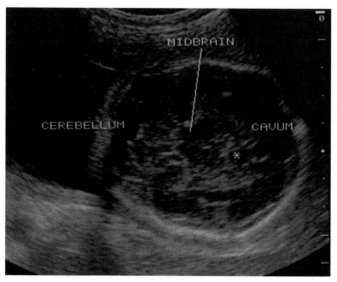

FIG. 4-7. The posterior fossa contains the symmetric, round cerebellar peduncles and the cisterna magna. The cisterna magna is an echolucent, crescent-shaped area between the cerebellum and the occipital bone.

monochorionic); or have some fusion of the fetal bodies (conjoint twins). Dizygotic twins will always be diamnionic, dichorionic. The placentas can be so closely juxtaposed in the uterus, however, that they can appear fused. The membrane boundary between diamnionic, dichorionic twins will be easily seen and should be relatively thick (when the origin from the placentas is examined, a "widow's peak" appearance of the two chorions will be seen) (Fig. 4-8) If twins in dichorionic, diamniotic twins are phenotypically of opposite gender, dizygotic twinning can be inferred. In these cases, the intervening membranes are made up of two layers of amnion and two layers of chorion, resulting in the thick membrane. Like-gender diamnionic, dichorionic twins could be either mono- or dizygotic.

A thin, wispy membrane and a common placenta indicates monochorionic, diamnionic twins. Late in pregnancy, or in the so-called stuck twin phenomenon, the intervening membrane made up of only two layers of amnion can be extremely difficult to visualize. Because the perinatal mortality and management of monoamnionic twins is so high relative to diamnionic twins, the distinction is an important one.

Any suspected deviation from normal fetal anatomy should be confirmed. This may simply require repeat scanning later in the day to obtain a more optimal fetal position, further efforts to look at more detailed images of the anatomy, perhaps trying endovaginal sonographs, or referral to a center in which the doctors are qualified to do a more thorough fetal examination. It is critical to recall that, if there is a birth defect present, there is a high probability that others are present and that karyotype analysis should be considered. In addition, the greatest known

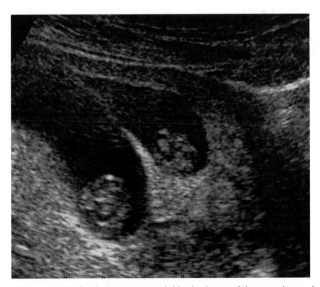

FIG. 4-8. The widow's peak of echolucent material in the base of the membrane between these two first trimester embryos suggests that these are diamniotic, dichorionic twins.

risk of prenatal ultrasound is false-positive diagnosis with the parental anxiety that it engenders and the possibility of elective termination of what is actually a normal fetus.

SUMMARY

Each clinician must decide upon the indications for requesting an obstetrical ultrasound. An understanding of the risk factors, etiologies, and clinical correlates with fetal anomalies and growth disturbances will aid in choosing the intensity with which the fetus is scrutinized. The content of even a basic ultrasound, however, should include an overview of the fetal anatomy, as outlined by ACOG and AIUM. Relying on these guidelines will improve the care of patients and increase the value of obstetric sonography.

FURTHER READING

American College of Gynecologists Technical Bulletin #187, December, 1993.

Benacerraf, BR. Who should be performing fetal ultrasound? [editorial] *Ultrasound Obstet Gynecol* 1993; 3:1–2.

Consensus Development Conference. DHHS Publication/NIH Publication No. 86-667. Bethesda, Maryland: National Institutes of Health, 1984.

Ewigman BG, Crane JP, Frigoletto FD, LeFevre ML, *et al*. Effect of prenatal ultrasound screening of perinatal outcome. *N Engl J Med* 1993;329:821–76.

Filly RA, Cardoza JD, Goldstein RB, Barkovich AJ. Detection of fetal central nervous system anomalies: a practical level of effort for a routine sonogram. *Radiology* 1989;172(2):403–8.

Guidelines for Performance of the Antepartum Obstetrical Ultrasound Examination. American Institute of Ultrasound in Medicine, Rockville, Maryland, 1991.

LeFevre ML, Bain RP, Ewigman BG, Frigoletto FD, *et al*. A randomized trial of prenatal ultrasonographic screening: impact on maternal management and outcome. *Am J Obstet Gynecol* 1993;169:483–9.

5

Fetal Biometry

While Dorland's *Illustrated Medical Dictionary* defines biometry as the "mathematical analysis of biologic data," in obstetric sonography it generally refers to the measurement of fetal body parts. Appropriate, precise fetal measurements can help to answer three basic questions: What is the approximate gestational age of this pregnancy? Is this fetus growing at a normal rate? Is there symmetry in growth of the fetus; if not, what may have caused the asymmetry?

In general, the size of fetal body parts correlates with gestational age. Among most populations, fetal size as a function of gestational age is similar during the first two trimesters of pregnancy, while among third-trimester fetuses there is an increasing variance of growth between normal, same-gestational-age fetuses. Consequently, the range of error in assigning gestational age increases later in pregnancy. Importantly, **the earliest competent examination is the best estimator of gestational age, and gestational age should not be reassigned if a third-trimester scan differs from an earlier one.**

Contemporary science and medicine relies heavily on numbers, but it is critical not to be entranced by the ability of the computer in the ultrasound unit to report a measurement in hundredths of a millimeter or tenths of a week. The product of the process of imaging and measuring a fetus becomes a clinical tool for caring for the patient; differences of tenths of a millimeter or less-than-a-week estimation of gestation have no role in clinical management. The axial resolution of most ultrasound transducers is 1 millimeter, not a hundredth of one.

Of the many charts that have been produced, the majority were obtained from scanning women with certain clinical dating parameters. The range of error in clinically dated pregnancies is about plus-or-minus 2 weeks; therefore, ultrasound dating cannot be more precise than the dating of the populations from which they were derived. Some charts are now appearing generated from early scans on pregnancies resulting from assisted reproduction technologies, but there is some question about whether early embryonic growth in such pregnancies is the same as those from spontaneous pregnancies. In sum, there will remain a range of error in the prediction of gestational age from all ultrasound biometry and, to appropriately use data obtained from ultrasound, we must understand these potential sources of error.

Hadlock and Ott demonstrated that, by measuring multiple parameters in the same fetus and averaging the gestational ages associated with those measurements, the composite gestational age obtained is more accurate than any single dimension. Since there is a plethora of charts with normal measurements ranging from head diameters and circumferences to long bones, to ear and foot measurements, it is important to choose a combination of measurements that are practical to obtain and that help to answer the clinical questions. The measurements you choose will depend in part on the trimester of the pregnancy in question, the time devoted for the scan, and which charts are easily available (some of which will be stored in the computer in the ultrasound unit). Whichever you choose, make sure that your techniques match those used to generate the chart. By obtaining the correct scanplanes and using appropriate landmarks to guide cursor placement, systematic error will be decreased.

Technical error can be minimized by making at least two measurements of each structure and scrutinizing them for consistency: each linear measurement should be within 1 mm of the other, and each circumference measurement should be within 10% of the other. If your repeated measurements fall within these differences and you are using the appropriate scanplane and cursor placements, further measurements will not increase the accuracy.

Another source of error in fetal measurement is the inclusion of data from abnormal anatomy in assigning gestational age. For instance, if one is imaging a third-trimester fetus with macrocrania secondary to hydrocephalus, the head measurements should not be included when assigning gestational age. Likewise, the abdominal circumference measurement in a fetus with intrauterine growth restriction or femur length in the case of a skeletal dysplasia should not be used in assigning gestational age. Significant discrepancies (such as the short femur associated with some aneuploidies or the biparietal diameter (BPD) that is small for gestational age in the second-trimester fetus with open spina bifida) should not be ignored, because they can be a clue to the presence of abnormal anatomy. It is obvious that the measurements obtained must be considered individually before averaging them to calculate the gestational age.

BIOMETRY AT WORK

The way that precise measurement of the fetus will work for you will depend on the clinical situation. As Rossavik stated, the "validity of any dating procedure, whether based on growth or dating equations or on one or two examinations, depends upon its ability to differentiate those women who have wrong dates from those who do not." To try to assign gestational age on the basis of ultrasound, the fetal age is considered the dependent variable and the fetal size is the independent variable, and the provider interprets the age based on the measurements. On the other hand, if one is trying to decide whether the fetus is growing normally, the fetal age is considered the independent variable, and the fetal size, the dependent one. Thus, in a patient with uncertain dates and late onset of prenatal care in whom a scan is being done for determining the gestational age, it will be very difficult to determine on the basis of a single scan whether the fetus is appropriately grown, since the independent variable (fetal age) is unknown. Accurate knowledge of fetal growth requires a firm knowledge of gestational age, either by sure clinical dating and an ultrasound or serial scans, assuming the first establishes the gestational age. If the provider relies on serial scans for the assessment of fetal growth, these scans should be at least 2 weeks apart. The difference between fetal measurements in a normally growing fetus in the third trimester are small enough that at least 2 weeks are necessary to escape potential technical errors and to define a growth abnormality.

Several authors have demonstrated that published charts, usually obtained from a homogeneous, well-dated population, are accurate when applied to different populations. Under ideal circumstances, however, each ultrasound unit will establish its own charts. If you find that published charts do not fit your technique or population, it is imperative that you do this.

FIRST TRIMESTER

Biometry in the first trimester has traditionally included a measurement of the size of the gestational sac if the scan is done prior to visibility of the embryo, followed by the crown-rump length (CRL) later on. The addition of transvaginal sonography with better visualization of the later first-trimester fetus has allowed for more precise visualization, and thus measurement, of the embryonic body. Kusterman reported on scans of 270 clinically dated pregnancies and was able to demonstrate that the CRL was obtainable in more than 80% of embryos at less than or equal to 11 weeks; BPD, head circumference (HC), and femur length (FL) were obtainable in over 80% of embryos at 10, 14, and 12 weeks, respectively. Kusterman's data show that most of the measurements correlated more with the CRL than with the estimated gestational age, suggesting either a wide range in the days of conception or genetic/environmental factors that modulate embryonic growth even this early in pregnancy.

The gestational sac measurement should be obtained in 3 dimensions (Fig. 5-1). The cursors are placed on the inside of the sac, at the border of the sac with the underlying uterus, and a mean sac size is obtained (Table 5-1).

A CRL is more difficult to obtain than it should seem (Fig. 5-2). It is possible to measure the CRL until about 12–14 weeks, at which time the embryo begins to curl making the CRL nonlinear and decreasing the accuracy of the measurement. The image should be frozen with the embryo seen in sagittal view with a clear image of the crown all the way to the caudal end of the fetus, excluding the extremities and the yolk sac (Table 5-2A,B).

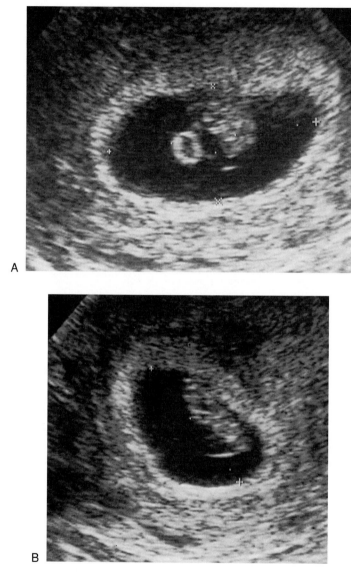

FIG. 5-1. A,B: The mean gestational sac measurement is obtained by averaging the three inner-to-inner diameters of the sac, taken at 90 degrees to each other.

TABLE 5-1. *Mean gestational sac diameters (mm)*

	Hellman		Grisolia	
Weeks	Mean	5th	Mean	95th
5	10	—	10	20
6	17	6	16	26
7	24	13	23	33
8	31	19	29	39
9	38	25	35	45
10	45	30	40	50
11	52	35	45	55
12	59	40	50	60

Second and Third Trimester

In contrast to the first-trimester embryo for which there are few choices for accurate measurement, we are faced with too many choices in the later trimesters. By choosing to measure the fetal head, abdomen, and a long bone, however, it is possible to reduce the many errors that are possible in fetal sonography.

The **biparietal diameter** (BPD) is one of the most commonly measured distances. It can be affected by fetal position, low amniotic fluid volumes, and intracranial pathology (Fig. 5-3).

The correct level of the fetal cranium for the measurement of the BPD is achieved when the scanplane is perpendicular to the midline of the fetal skull in

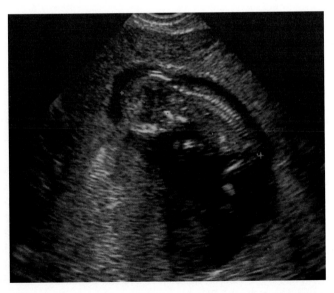

FIG. 5-2. The crown-rump length is the maximum linear measurement from the top of the cranium to the gluteal region.

TABLE 5-2A. *Crown-rump length (CRL) associated with known gestational age[a]*

	CRL		
Weeks	5th	Mean	95th
5	1	3	5
6	2	6	10
7	4	10	16
8	8	16	24
9	12	23	34
10	18	31	44
11	26	40	54
12	33	50	67

[a] From Grisolia F, Milano V, Pilu G, *et al.* Biometry of early sonography with transvaginal sonography. *Ultrasound Obstet Gynecol* 1993;3:403–11.

TABLE 5-2B. *Gestational age associated with known CRL[a]*

CRL	Days
8	49.1
15	57.0
23	63.2
32	70.5
42	77.4
54	84.2

[a] From Daya S. Accuracy of gestational age estimation by means of fetal crown-rump length measurement. *Am J Obstet Gynecol* 1993;168:903–8.

an occipitofrontal orientation just above the orbits. This is the largest plane of the fetal head, and it provides an oval skull outline with a centered midline and symmetric parietal bone curvature.

The easiest approach to develop such an image is to align the transducer with the fetal spine, slide the transducer cranially until the head is seen, and then turn it 90 degrees. An inappropriate coronal scanplane will produce a more circular outline of the fetal cranium, if it is a dorsal coronal view, or will demonstrate fetal orbits, if it is a ventral coronal view. Once the appropriate oval cranial shape is seen, the angle of the scanplane should be adjusted to center the midline. The transducer is then moved up or down to produce the largest oval cranial outline. If intracranial anatomy is visible, the cavum septum pellucidum and the thalami are usually seen. The correct BPD is the largest transcranial diameter perpendic-

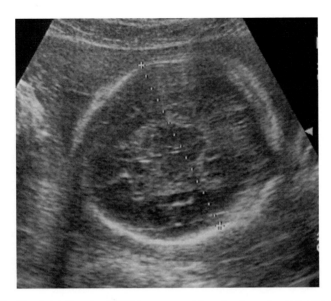

FIG. 5-3. The biparietal diameter (BPD) is measured from leading edge to leading edge of the skull, in a scanplane that includes the cavum septum pellucidum and thalami but omits the cerebellum.

ular to the midline in this plane. The measurement is made from the leading edge (closest to transducer) of the proximal skull table to the leading edge of the distal table.

The occipitofrontal diameter (OFD) is obtained on the same image, measuring in the midline from the front to the back of the skull, from outer to outer edge of the bone (Fig. 5-4).

Head circumference (HC) measurements can be helpful when the head shape is abnormal, as in the dolichocephalic fetus. Importantly, the circumference is calculated from the OFD and the transverse diameter of the skull at the level of the BPD but including the full diameter of the skull, from outer to outer skull edge. If you use the linear measurements of the BPD and OFD, it will systematically underestimate the head circumference, since the traditional BPD measures leading edge to leading edge. The ellipse function of many ultrasound machines allows the sonographer to measure the full circumference of the skull but essentially only averages the two diameters and then calculates the circumference (Fig. 5-5) (Table 5-3).

The fetal long bone most commonly measured is the fetal **femur.** The same principles apply, however, in any long-bone measurement. The image should show a homogeneously dense bone, with shadowing seen behind it (Fig. 5-6). The edges of the bone should be crisply seen. Imaging the femur may be accomplished by longitudinally aligning the transducer with the spine, sliding it to the

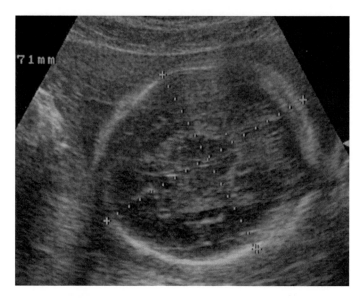

FIG. 5-4. The same image is used for a head circumference measurement as for a BPD. The head circumference includes the entire head, therefore the cursors are placed from leading edge to trailing edge for the transverse head measurement and outer table to outer table for the occipitofrontal diameters.

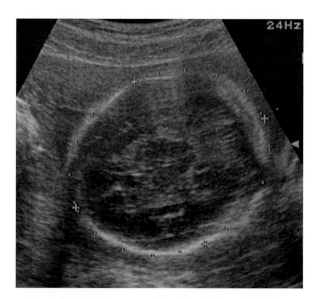

FIG. 5-5. The head circumference may be measured using the ellipse function. The ellipse should outline the outer margins of the skull.

TABLE 5-3. *Cranial measurements; biparietal diameter and head circumference*

Menstrual age (wk)	Hadlock BPD (cm) ± SD[a]	Chitty BPD (mm)[b]	Chitty HC (plotted)[b]		
			3rd	50th	97th
12	2.10 ± 0.13	1.93 ± 0.15	57.5	69.6	81.6
13	2.27 ± 0.06	2.19 ± 0.16	71.2	83.7	96.2
14	2.70 ± 0.14	2.73 ± 0.21	84.8	97.7	110.7
15	2.98 ± 0.16	2.95 ± 0.22	98.2	111.5	124.9
16	3.30 ± 0.13	3.36 ± 0.23	111.3	125.1	138.9
17	3.36 ± 0.18	3.58 ± 0.29	124.2	138.5	152.7
18	3.95 ± 0.15	4.05 ± 0.24	136.9	151.6	166.2
19	4.28 ± 0.24	4.34 ± 0.23	149.3	164.4	179.5
20	4.56 ± 0.24	4.52 ± 0.27	161.5	177.0	192.5
21	4.84 ± 0.21	4.91 ± 0.28	173.3	189.3	205.3
22	5.21 ± 0.22	5.21 ± 0.33	184.9	201.3	217.7
23	5.48 ± 0.27	5.56 ± 0.38	196.1	213.0	229.8
24	5.86 ± 0.21	5.84 ± 0.33	207.0	224.6	241.6
25	6.15 ± 0.17	6.16 ± 0.32	217.6	235.3	253.0
26	6.35 ± 0.25	6.38 ± 0.37	227.8	246.0	264.1
27	6.69 ± 0.19	6.84 ± 0.33	237.7	256.3	274.9
28	7.01 ± 0.16	7.18 ± 0.34	247.2	266.2	285.2
29	7.20 ± 0.17	7.48 ± 0.20	256.2	275.7	295.1
30	7.45 ± 0.25	7.70 ± 0.31	264.9	284.8	304.6
31	7.59 ± 0.19	7.85 ± 0.31	273.1	293.4	313.7
32	7.86 ± 0.26	8.13 ± 0.33	280.9	301.6	322.4
33	8.16 ± 0.23	8.24 ± 0.43	288.2	309.4	330.6
34	8.33 ± 0.16	8.48 ± 0.29	295.1	316.7	338.3
35	8.69 ± 0.21	8.67 ± 0.38	301.4	323.5	345.5
36	8.79 ± 0.17	8.85 ± 0.42	307.3	329.8	352.3
37	8.90 ± 0.24	9.02 ± 0.45	312.7	335.6	358.5
38	9.14 ± 0.27	9.19 ± 0.40	317.5	340.8	364.2
39	9.26 ± 0.43	9.21 ± 0.35	321.8	345.6	369.4
40	9.44 ± 0.30	9.49 ± 0.44	325.5	349.7	374.0

[a] From Hadlock FP, Deter RL, Harris RB, Park SK. Fetal biparietal diameter: a critical reevaluation of the relation to menstrual age by means of real-time ultrasound. *J Ultrasound Med* 1982;1:97–104.
[b] From Chitty LS, Altman DG, Henderson A, Campbell S. Charts of fetal size: 2. head measurements. *Br J Obstet Gynecol* 1994;101:35:43.
Wk, week; BPD, biparietal diameter; HC, head circumference.

caudal end of the fetus, and rotating the transducer slowly toward the ventral aspect of the fetus until the femur comes into view. Alternatively, the transducer may be placed transverse to the fetal spine and moved caudally until a portion of one femur is seen transversely, within the usually flexed thigh. Often, only a fraction of a femur will be seen at first, and rotation of the transducer is necessary to capture a greater length of the bone. Rotation and slight angling will convince the operator that the entire length has been captured. The image must then be frozen and the length from end to end parallel to the shaft measured. Acoustical shadows are helpful in discriminating an occasional extension artifact from real bone.

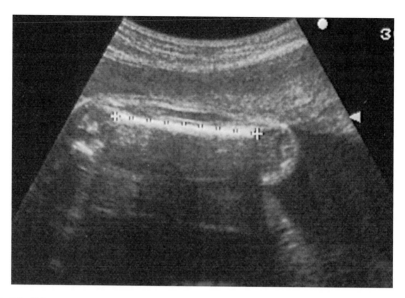

FIG. 5-6. When obtaining an image of a long bone for measurement, try to have the bone as perpendicular as possible to the ultrasound beam. The bone should be homogeneously dense and the bone ends should be clearly defined.

The femur length shows less variation in late pregnancy than does the head measurement (Table 5-4).

The **abdominal circumference (AC)** is an important measurement, especially when one is trying to judge fetal growth. Because the liver is the site of storage of glycogen and is the largest abdominal organ, fetuses with inadequate glycogen stores (due to nutritional deprivation) will have relatively small abdomens and therefore their AC measurement should be discordantly small relative to the head measurements (the so-called brain-sparing effect). Unfortunately, the AC is the one commonly performed measurement that has the worst reproducibility. This makes sense in that the abdomen is entirely soft tissue and is deformable by too much transducer pressure, fetal positioning, and myomas. Nonetheless, it is an important measurement to obtain well, because it is a component of all estimates of fetal weights. The abdominal circumference should be obtained in a plane perpendicular to the spine, at a level in which the stomach is visible, as is the linear portion of the umbilical vein as it passes through the liver (Fig. 5-7). This portion of the vein should be approximately one third of the way toward the middle of the abdomen from the anterior abdominal wall. Importantly, the fetal kidneys and umbilical cord insertion should not be visible. Since the ribs are oriented oblique to the perpendicular, multiple cross-sections of ribs should be visible in the ap-

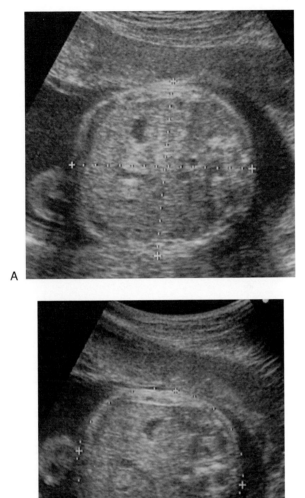

A

B

FIG. 5-7. The abdominal circumference (AC) is measured in a scanplane transverse to the fetal spine with the stomach and umbilical vein both visible. The AC can be calculated by (7**A**) calculating a mean abdominal diameter and using the formula circumference AC = $d1 + dz \times {}^{\pi}/_{2}$ or by (7**B**) using the ellipse mechanism.

TABLE 5-4. *Fetal long bone measurements*

Weeks	Hadlock[a] femur mm	Merz[b] femur mm	Kim-Kern[b] humerus mm
12	8		
13	11	11	10
14	15	13	12
15	18	15	14
16	21	19	17
17	24	22	20
18	27	25	23
19	30	28	26
20	33	31	29
21	36	35	32
22	39	36	33
23	42	40	37
24	44	42	38
25	47	46	42
26	49	48	43
27	52	49	45
28	54	53	47
29	56	53	48
30	58	56	50
31	61	60	53
32	63	61	54
33	65	64	56
34	66	66	58
35	68	67	59
36	70	70	60
37	72	72	61
38	73	74	64
39	75	76	65
40	76	77	66

[a] From Hadlock FP, Harris RB, Deter RL, Park SK. Fetal femur length as a predictor of menstrual age: sonographically measured. *AJR* 1982;138:875–8.

[b] From Mertz E, Kim-Kern M, Pehl S. Ultrasonic mensuration of fetal limb bones in the second and third trimesters. *J Clin Ultrasound* 1987;15:175–83.

propriate scanplane. Measurement is made by placing the cursors on the skin edge. If the circumference is to be calculated from the mean diameters, obtain two diameters, both of which cross the midpoint of the abdomen and are at right angles to each other. This is most easily obtained by measuring transverse diameters that are in the anterior-posterior orientation, intersecting with the fetal spine and the diameter at 90 degrees to that. However, late in pregnancy, a large fetus may not be oriented in such a way that the deep skin edge is visible for these standard measurements, but another set of perpendicular measurements are possible. Repeat measurements of the AC should be within 10% of each other for reliability (Table 5-5).

TABLE 5-5. *Fetal abdominal circumference and estimation of gestational age*

Weeks	Hadlock,[a] 1982 mean (cm) ± SD		Hadlock,[b] 1990 mean (cm)
15	9.87	0.53	—
16	10.47	1.14	—
17	11.36	0.86	—
18	12.77	0.83	—
19	13.58	1.43	—
20	15.49	1.29	—
21	15.82	1.00	15.9
22	16.91	1.38	17.0
23	18.72	1.81	18.2
24	19.72	1.01	19.3
25	21.36	0.97	20.4
26	22.08	1.25	21.5
27	23.09	0.97	22.6
28	24.66	1.55	23.6
29	25.00	1.08	24.7
30	25.21	1.32	25.7
31	26.59	1.38	26.7
32	27.15	0.87	27.7
33	28.90	1.37	28.7
34	29.78	1.36	29.6
35	30.46	1.23	30.5
36	31.22	1.15	31.5
37	32.95	1.46	32.4
38	33.93	1.39	33.2
39	34.51	1.49	34.1
40	34.91	1.29	35.0

[a] From Hadlock FP, Peter RL, Harris RB, Park SK. Fetal abdominal circumference as a predictor of menstrual age. *AJR* 1982;139:367–70.
[b] From Hadlock FP, Harris RB, Shah YP, Sharman RS, Park SK. Sonographic fetal growth standards; are current data applicable to a racially mixed population? *J Ultrasound Med* 1990;9:157–60.

OTHER MEASUREMENTS

In addition to the BPD, HC, AC, and FL, other fetal parts can be measured. Some authors have suggested that **transverse cerebellar diameters** (TCD) are useful to screen for intrauterine growth delay, as the fetal brain sparing effect will allow for continued normal growth of the posterior fossa contents, despite failure of the fetal abdomen and long bones to continue to grow (Fig. 5-8). It is appealing to measure an intracranial structure for this purpose, since the fetal cranium could be distorted if there is significant oligohydramnios, while the cerebellum

TABLE 5-6. *Miscellaneous fetal measurementss*

Weeks	Sherer[a] Sacrum (cm)	Lettieri[b] Ear length (mm)	Platt[c] Foot length (cm)
15	1.4	8	1.78
16	1.5	9	2.08
17	1.6	11	2.39
18	1.7	12	2.70
19	1.8	13	3.01
20	1.9	14	3.32
21	2.0	16	3.62
22	2.1	17	3.93
23	2.2	18	4.24
24	2.3	19	4.55
25	2.4	21	4.86
26	2.5		5.16
27	2.6		5.47
28	2.7		5.78
29	2.7		
30	3.0		
31	3.1		
32	3.2		
33	3.3		
34	3.4		
35	3.5		
36	3.6		
37	3.7		
38	3.8		
39	3.9		
40	4.0		

[a] From Sherer DM, Abramowicz JS, Plessinger MA, Woods JR. Fetal sacral length in the ultrasonographic assessment of gestational age. *Am J Obstet Gynecol* 1993;168:626–33.

[b] From Lettieri L, Rodis JF, Vintzileos AM, Feeney L, Ciarleglio L, Caffrey A. Ear length in second-trimester aneuploid fetuses. *Obstet Gynecol* 1993;81:57–60.

[c] Platt LD, Medearis AL, DeVore GR, Horenstein JM, Carlson DE, Brar HS. Fetal foot length: relationship to menstrual age and fetal measurements in the second trimester. *Obstet Gynecol* 1988;71:526–31.

should not be changed by such distortion. Nonetheless, other authors dispute the usefulness of the cerebellum for this purpose.

Table 5-6 includes some of the published data on other body measurements. In the abnormal pregnancy, particularly one in which there is asymmetric growth or abnormal anatomy, making additional measurements may help to define the abnormality more clearly.

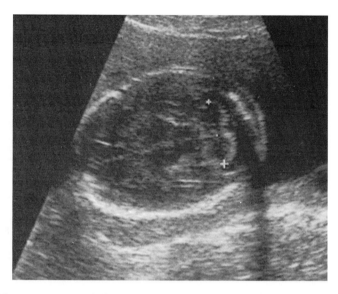

FIG 5-8. The transverse cerebellar diameter is measured at the widest part of the cerebellum at the level of the thalami and cavum septum pellucidum.

SUMMARY

Precise measurements of the fetus using a combination of parameters allows one to determine gestational age within a range of possibilities, to assess the normalcy of fetal growth, and to screen for some birth defects. It is critical that measurements be made in appropriate scanplanes, with proper cursor placement, and with repetition of the measurements to assure precision.

FURTHER READING

Chitty LS, Altman DG, Henderson A, Campbell S. Charts of fetal size: 2. head measurements. *Br J Obstet Gynaecol* 1994;101:35–43.

Daya S. Accuracy of gestational age estimation by means of fetal crown-rump length measurement. *Am J Obstet Gynecol* 1993;168:903–8.

Friel JP, ed. Dorland's *Illustrated Medical Dictionary,* 26th ed. Philadelphia: W.B. Saunders Company, 1980:169.

Goldstein I, Reece EA, Pilu G, Bovicelli L, Hobbins JC. Cerebellar measurements with ultrasonography in the evaluation of fetal growth and development. *Am J Obstet Gynecol* 1987;156:1065–9.

Grisolia F, Milano V, Pilu G, *et al.* Biometry of early sonography with transvaginal sonography. *Ultrasound Obstet Gynecol* 1993;3:403–11.

Hadlock FP, Deter RL, Harris RB, Park SK. Fetal biparietal diameter: a critical re-evaluation of the relation to menstrual age by means of real-time ultrasound. *J Ultrasound Med* 1982;1:97–104.

Hadlock FP, Deter RL, Harris RB, Park SK. Fetal abdominal circumference as a predictor of menstrual age. *AJR* 1982;139:367–70.

Hadlock FP, Harris RB, Martinex-Poyer J. How accurate is second trimester fetal dating? *J Ultrasound Med* 1991;10:557–61.

Hadlock FP, Harris RB, Shah YP, Sharman RS, Park SK. Sonographic fetal growth standards; are current data applicable to a racially mixed population? *J Ultrasound Med* 1990;9:157–60.

Hadlock FP, Harris RB, Deter RL, Park SK. Fetal femur length as a predictor of menstrual age: sonographically measured. *AJR* 1982;138:875–8.

Hellman LM, Kobayashi M, Fillisti L, Lavenhar M, Cromb E. Growth and development of the human fetus prior to the twentieth week of gestation. *Am J Obstet Gynecol* 1969;103:789–800.

Hill LM, Guzick D, Hixson J, Peterson CS, Rivello DM. Composite assessment of gestational age: a comparison of institutionally derived and published regression equations. *Am J Obstet Gynecol* 1992;166:551–5.

Hill LM, Guzick D, Rivello D, Hixson J, Peterson C. The transverse cerebellar diameter cannot be used to assess gestational age in the small for gestational age fetus. *Obstet Gynecol* 1990;75:329–33.

Kusterman A, Zorzoli A, Spagnolo D, Nicolini U. Transvaginal sonography for fetal measurement in early pregnancy. *Br J Obstet Gynaecol* 1992;99:38–42.

Lettieri L, Rodis JF, Vintzileos AM, Feeney L, Ciarleglio L, Craffey A. Ear length in second-trimester aneuploid fetuses. *Obstet Gynecol* 1993;81:57–60.

Merz E, Kim-Kern M, Pehl S. Ultrasonic mensuration of fetal limb bones in the second and third trimesters. *J Clin Ultrasound* 1987;15:175–83.

Ott WJ. Accurate gestational dating. *Obstet Gynecol* 1985;66:311–5.

Platt LD, Medearis AL, DeVore GR, Horenstein JM, Carlson DE, Brar HS. Fetal foot length: relationship to menstrual age and fetal measurements in the second trimester. *Obstet Gynecol* 1988;71:526–31.

Rossavik IK, Fishburne JI. Conceptional age, menstrual age, and ultrasound age: a second-trimester comparison of pregnancies of known conception date with pregnancies dated from the last menstrual period. *Obstet Gynecol* 1989;73:243–9.

Reece EA, Goldstein I, Pilu G, Hobbins JC. Fetal cerebellar growth unaffected by intrauterine growth retardation: a new parameter for prenatal diagnosis. *Am J Obstet Gynecol* 1987;157:632–8.

Sherer DM, Abramowicz JS, Plessinger MA, Woods JR. Fetal sacral length in the ultrasonographic assessment of gestational age. *Am J Obstet Gynecol* 1993;168:626–33.

6

Estimated Fetal Weight in the Case of Prematurity, Intrauterine Growth Restriction, and Macrosomia

Intrauterine growth restriction (IUGR) and macrosomia both impose significant perinatal morbidity and mortality burdens on affected infants. Both conditions are defined by birthweight above or below certain levels and often characterized by certain recognizable biometric asymmetries. Accurate estimation of fetal weight (EFW), therefore, is an important clinical capability that may anticipate these conditions and allow more appropriate clinical management. Furthermore, perinatal management of ruptured membranes, preterm labor, and many other complications of pregnancy that may require delivery during the early viable period benefit from an accurate knowledge of fetal weight since more accurate parameters of fetal viability may be unavailable.

The desired result of the management process is to deliver the healthiest neonate, not just to make the diagnosis of a growth disorder. The practical limits of precision of EFW must be incorporated into clinical judgment, and an assessment of fetal condition within the context of growth and gestational age are both fundamental to appropriate use of EFW.

CLINICAL ESTIMATION

Traditional estimation of fetal weight by manual palpation results in an EFW with wide variance. Rupture of membranes, oligohydramnios, malpresentation, uterine anomalies, deep pelvic engagement, twins, polyhydramnios, and other clinical conditions all add to the inaccuracy of manual estimation of fetal weight. The measurement in centimeters from the pubic symphysis to the top of the fundus between 20 and 35 weeks approximates the gestational age in weeks. If the fundal height is 3 or more cm greater or less than expected, inference about dates or fetal growth may be made, and ultrasound may be used to clarify the apparent clinical discrepancy.

ULTRASOUND ESTIMATION OF FETAL WEIGHT

The earliest method for the estimation of fetal weight using ultrasonic biometry was reported in 1973 by Campbell and was based only on abdominal circumference. Derived from a largely uncomplicated population delivering normal infants, the system showed an accuracy of about ±15%. However, when applied to complicated pregnancies involving infants with any significant asymmetry of growth, accuracy was diminished.

In 1977, a system using biparietal diameter and abdominal circumference was reported by Warsoff with a variance of about ±10% (1 SD). This mathematical relationship between fetal dimensions and birthweight was based

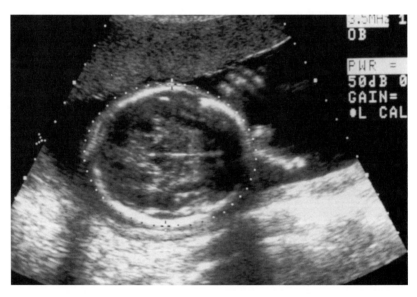

FIG. 6-1. The biparietal diameter (BPD) or head circumference (HC) used to estimate fetal weight is identical to the dimensions used for dating. The HC illustrated here shows the placement of the ellipse cursors at the outer edge of the skull table.

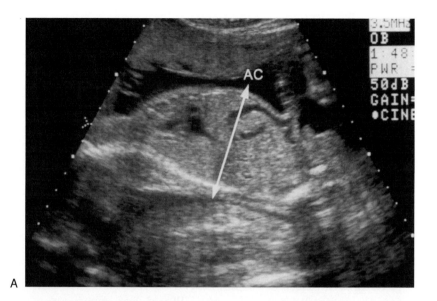

A

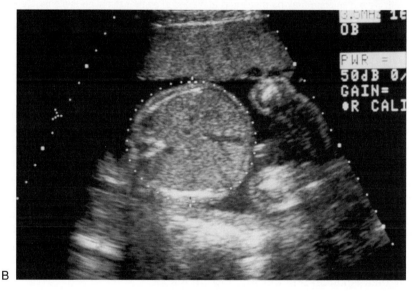

B

FIG. 6-2. A: This sagittal sonogram of the fetus shows the approximate placement of the transverse plane at the level of the umbilical vein deep in the liver mass below the diaphragm. **B:** Transverse placement of the scanplane at the position shown in A should produce an image similar to this with the umbilical vein located in the fetal sagittal midline, and the stomach to the fetal right side.

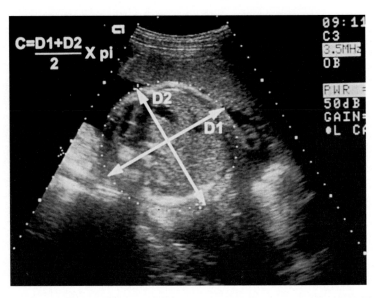

FIG. 6-3. Two diameters may be measured and used in some estimation systems. Typically, one diameter is the sagittal midline skin to skin, and the other, perpendicular to it. However, if the abdomen is noncircular, the examiner is most interested in the long axis and the short axis diameters regardless of the anatomy.

on a logarithmic transformation that might be programmed into a hand-held computer, or the clinician could use published bivariant tables. The more dimensions used in any system, the more control of variance is expected especially in the case of the asymmetric fetus. Since 1977, numerous methodologies have been reported, most using biparietal diameter (BPD) (Fig. 6-1) and abdominal circumference (AC) (Fig. 6-2A,B) or mean abdominal diameter (MAD) (Fig. 6-3), some using femur length (FL) (Fig. 6-4) and abdominal circumference, and some using all three. A few research activities have used more dimensions than these but are of limited practical value, because the time needed to produce the raw data is burdensome and the calculation of the mathematical relationship, too complex.

Most current ultrasound machines incorporate one or more of the more recent weight estimation formulae into the obstetric software package in the machine. Some allow the user to program a preferred formula into the machine if the packaged method is not a favorite. Anyone who uses EFW in clinical practice needs to know which system is built into his or her machine and record experience with it to document the accuracy of the system being used.

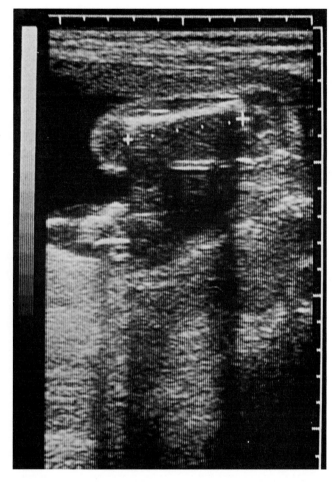

FIG. 6-4. The same femur length technique used for gestational age assessment is used for estimation of fetal weight. Measurement of the femur is illustrated here from metaphyseal plate to metaphyseal plate, parallel to the shaft.

THE BASIS

The theoretical basis of sonographic estimation of fetal weight is simply that the larger a fetus is, the larger most sonographic dimensions will be. As stated above, the more dimensions used, the more accurate the system is likely to be, but the more dimensions used, the less practical a system will be. No two systems

TABLE 6–1. *Selected EFW methodologies*

Formulas	Source
Log BW = −1.599 + 0.144(BPD) + 0.032(AC) − 0.111(BPD2 × AC)/1000	Warsof, 1977
Log BW = −1.792 + 0.166(BPD) + 0.046(AC) − 2.646(AC × BPD)/1000	Shepard, 1982
Log BW = 1.304 + 0.05281(AC) + 0.1938(FL) − 0.004(AC × FL)	Hadlock, 1984
ln BW = 0.143 X + 4.198 X = BPD + MAD + FL in cm	Rose and McCallum, 1987

demonstrate identical accuracy or precision, and every system works best for its original author. Virtually all practical current methods use AC or MAD plus one or more other dimensions, typically BPD, HC, or femur. Those that use three might be expected to produce the least variance in the case of complicated pregnancies, but, overall, none has proved to be of significance superiority (Table 6-1). In the case in which your equipment has no built-in capability, reference to tables is the practical alternative to complex mathematical formulae. The simplest method uses BPD, MAD, and FL (Table 6-2, Rose and McCallum).

TABLE 6–2. *Estimation of fetal weight using BPD, FL, and MAD*

X = BPD + MAD + FL					
X	EFW	X	EFW	X	EFW
14.0	493	19.5	1082	25.0	2376
14.5	529	20.0	1162	25.5	2552
15.0	569	20.5	1248	26.0	2741
15.5	611	21.0	1341	26.5	2944
16.0	656	21.5	1440	27.0	3162
16.5	705	22.0	1547	27.5	3397
17.0	757	22.5	1662	28.0	3648
17.5	813	23.0	1785	28.5	3919
18.0	873	23.5	1917	29.0	4209
18.5	938	24.0	1059	29.5	4521
19.0	1007	24.5	2212	30.0	4856

Modified from Rose BI, McCallum WD. A simplified method for estimating fetal weight using ultrasound measurements. *Obstet Gynecol* 1987;69:671.
BPD, biparietal diameter; FL, femur length; MAD, mean abdominal diameter; EFW, estimation of fetal weight.

ACCURACY

Current, practical systems all provide an EFW with a similar variance of about ± 8–10% (1 SD). Some might be a little better than this, others a bit worse, but all are close to this level. What this means is that the sonographic EFW will be within 10% of the actual birthweight 67% of the time (± 1 SD). If the user requires 95% confidence, than the range is as great as ± 20% (± 2 SD). Significantly asymmetric growth would diminish this level of accuracy.

Most methods are most accurate in the normally grown symmetric fetus and least accurate in the asymmetric IUGR fetus or the macrosomic infant because of asymmetric growth not reflected perfectly by the limited dimensions used. Proper technique is critical to achievement of even this level of precision. The abdominal circumference is the least reproducible and most variable of all dimensions, and care must be taken to produce an accurate AC.

EFW AND PERINATAL MANAGEMENT

In the case of premature rupture of membranes, premature labor, or other clinical complications that may require preterm delivery, optimal management may depend on an estimation of fetal weight. An assessment of fetal potential for survival, the benefits of intrapartum monitoring, the benefits of transfer to a center capable of managing extreme prematurity, and even the advisability of cesarean delivery for fetal indications may depend on an accurate estimate of fetal weight. Although some observers find that accurate gestational age is a better predictor of perinatal outcomes than weight alone, accurate gestational age data is often missing or unobtainable at the time management decisions are made and weight becomes the only objective estimator of potential for survival (Table 6-3).

Even an accurate EFW will, however, underestimate survivability in the case of the IUGR infant, and careful assessment of this possibility must be part of any clinical decision.

TABLE 6–3. *Age, weight, survival*

Weeks	BW	Survival %	Intact
22	500	0	0
24	650	17	9
26	900	51	41
28	1100	75	67
30	1400	87	81

From *ACOG Technical Bulletin* #13, 1989.

INTRAUTERINE GROWTH RESTRICTION (IUGR)

IUGR is defined as a birthweight under the tenth percentile for gestational age, judged from birthweight standards that are representative for the population in question. Birthweight standards recorded from a population at high altitude are not appropriate to judge growth for a population at low altitude.

It is clear that a sizable proportion of infants with a birthweight under the tenth percentile are small for familial constitutional reasons, and not because of toxic, genetic, or deprivational factors. Many small fetuses are not sick. However, the ability to discriminate one cause from another is often limited, and birthweight, or in the case of the fetus, EFW, is at least the most commonly used criterion for suspicion of the diagnosis.

It is clear that the larger a fetus is, the larger will be his or her dimensions. The widely varying accuracy and sensitivity in the detection of IUGR shown by several investigators for biparietal diameter by itself, serial biparietal diameters, abdominal circumference, and head circumference to abdominal circumference ratio probably reflect the variability in the growth characteristics of infants who are small because of deprivation compared with those infants who are small because of constitutional reasons.

In the case of the symmetrically small infant, all dimensions would be proportionately smaller than expected. If accurate clinical gestational age is available, the diagnosis of **symmetric IUGR** may be made. However, if clinical estimated gestational age (EGA) is suspect or unavailable, differentiation of symmetric IUGR from erroneous EGA may be impossible at a single examination.

In the case of **asymmetric IUGR,** typically the result of intrauterine deprivation or impaired uteroplacental function, the physiology of the fetal response to deprivation results in a "brain sparing" effect. Fetal cardiac output is reoriented to favor brain, coronary arteries, and adrenal glands. The result is normal or near normal brain growth late into a deprivational sequence of growth. Sequential surveillance of growth parameters over time may assist in the diagnosis of IUGR.

Single fetal dimensions, then, are limited in the diagnosis of IUGR. Abdominal circumference, small for dates in both symmetric and asymmetric IUGR, is expected to show the greatest diagnostic sensitivity but requires an accurate EGA to be useful.

Ratios of biparietal diameter or femur length to abdominal circumference that reflect asymmetries of growth show considerable utility with or without an accurate EGA, since abnormalities of these ratios at any age reflect the asymmetric growth associated with deprivation. Symmetric IUGR, however, may not be detected by such ratios. BPD to AC was the first ratio proposed, and more recently AC/FL has been examined. Therefore, assessment of abdominal circumference or combinations that include AC (such as certain biometric ratios) and estimated fetal weight show similar sensitivity and accuracy in the diagnosis of IUGR (Table 6-4).

TABLE 6–4. *Diagnosis of IUGR relative sensitivity*

Measure	Sensitivity (%)
Single BPD	49
Serial BPD	50
AC	83–100
HC/AC ratio	80
Femur length	20–45
Head/abdomen	70
EFW percentile	63–89
Femur/abdomen	57–63

TRANSCEREBELLAR DIAMETER

Recent reports of the correlation between transcerebellar diameter (TCD) and gestational age and the relative conservation of this relationship even in IUGR circumstances suggest a peculiar utility of this dimension in the discrimination of IUGR from misdated pregnancies. Initial reports of absolute preservation of TCD in all types of IUGR, however, appear optimistic. Other observers have found that, although TCD does sustain a normal growth pattern deep into a deprivational sequence, TCD is also small for dates in most symmetrically small fetuses.

TECHNIQUE

From the standard occipitofrontal BPD scanplane, generally at the level of the thalami, rotate the occipital heel of the transducer slightly caudally. The cerebellar hemispheres will become visible, although later in pregnancy they are not as visually distinct as earlier (Fig. 6-5). The ideal plane includes the cavum septum pellucidum, the brainstem/thalamus aggregate, and the cerebellar hemispheres. Measurement includes both hemispheres. Reference to a chart or table is necessary because no machines are currently programmed with this information (Table 6-5).

TABLE 6–5. *Relationship of transcerebellar diameter (TCD) to gestational age*

TCD (mm)	Gestational age (weeks)	TCD (mm)	Gestational age (weeks)
14	15	34	29
16	17	36	30
18	18	38	31
20	20	40	32
22	21	42	33
24	22	44	34
26	24	46	35
28	25	48	36
30	26	50	37
32	28	52	38

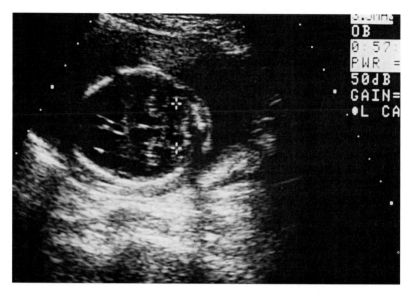

FIG. 6-5. Slight rotation of the occipital heel of the transducer from the typical BPD plane will bring the posterior fossa into view. The transcerebellar diameter is measured from the outer edge of one hemisphere to the outer edge of the other.

ESTIMATION OF FETAL WEIGHT AND IUGR

Since IUGR is defined on a weight basis, an accurate knowledge of fetal weight is the ideal element of the diagnosis (Table 6-6). Furthermore, IUGR is the result of a variety of etiologies including constitutional, teratogenic/genetic, infectious, and deprivational factors. These may produce a growth pattern that is either early or late in onset and either symmetric or asymmetric in pattern. The serial tracking of various fetal biometric parameters, as well as the analysis of the symmetry of these parameters may aid in detection and management (Fig. 6-6A–D).

TABLE 6–6. *10th, 50th, and 90th percentiles for EFW (in grams)*

Gestational age	10th percentile	50th percentile	90th percentile
28	1004	1210	1416
30	1294	1559	1824
32	1621	1953	2285
34	1973	2377	2781
36	2335	2813	3291
38	2686	3236	3786
40	3004	3619	4234

Modified from Hadlock FP, Harrist RB, Martinez-Poyer J. *In utero* anlaysis of fetal growth: a sonographic weight standard. *Radiology* 1991;181(1):129–33.

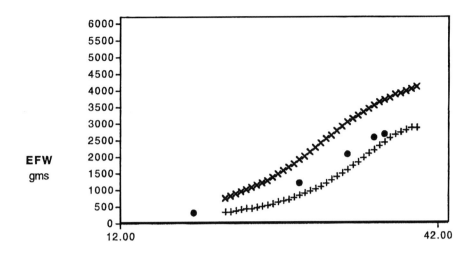

A

Clinical MA In Weeks

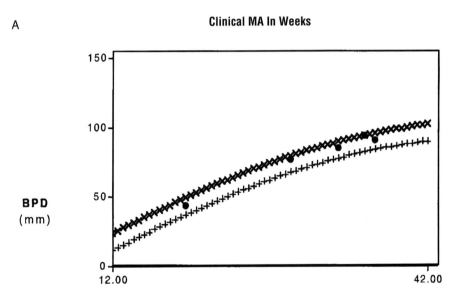

B   **Clinical MA In Weeks**

FIG. 6-6. A: Sequential EFW in the case of IUGR shows the EFW approaching the 10th percentile. **B:** Sequential BPD tracking, however, shows this measure remaining well within normal
limits.

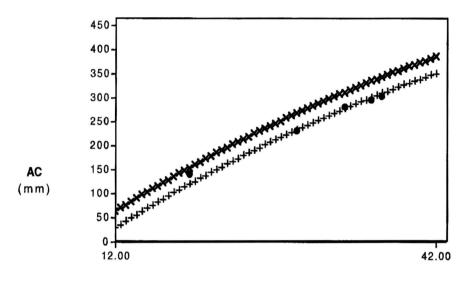

C

Clinical MA In Weeks

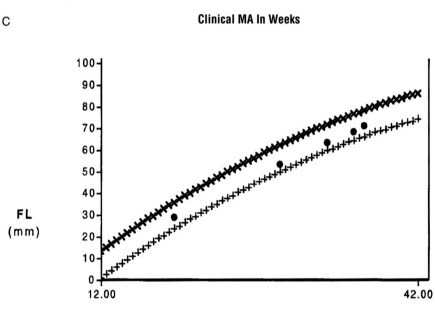

D

Clinical MA In Weeks

FIG. 6-6 *(Continued.)* **C:** In this case, only AC mirrors the EFW in falling from the normal growth curve. **D:** FL remains within the normal range.

TABLE 6–7. *Hypothetical clinical circumstances*

EFW	AFV	EGA	NST	MANAGEMENT
<10TH%	NL	?	R	Serial EFW/Surveillance
<10TH%	NL	<36W	R	Same
<10TH%	NL	>36W	R	Assess for delivery
<10TH%	OLIG	<36W	R	Close OBS/DEL if distress
<10TH%	OLIG	>36W	NR	Assess for delivery

EFW, estimation of fetal weight; AFV, amnionic fluid volume; EGA, estimated gestational age; NST, nonstress test; R, reactive; NR, non-reactive; OBS/DEL, observation/delivery.

Sonographic EFW has shown a diagnostic sensitivity of up to 90% with a positive predictive value of 60%. Although a 40% false-positive rate may seem high since the clinical response to the diagnosis in the preterm gestation is close fetal surveillance rather than immediate delivery, the benefits of high sensitivity may outweigh a false-positive rate.

Serial tracking of BPD, AC, and EFW may allow discrimination of IUGR of deprivational cause from IUGR of intrinsic fetal pathology such as genetic or infectious causes. In the fetus with near normal growth of BPD but AC growth dropping away from the normal growth curve, asymmetric IUGR may be suspected. Regardless, EFW has become the main sonographic parameter of fetal growth.

A number of authors have recognized the correlation between maternal risk factors, oligohydramnios, low EFW, and IUGR. Scoring systems have been proposed that produce numeric scores as a result of these observations. It is doubtful, however, that any numerical score will replace considered clinical judgement (Table 6-7). If the nonstress test (NST) is reactive with normal fluid with unsure dates or remote from term, expectant management with careful fetal surveillance is appropriate. Near term with oligohydramnios, even with a reactive NST, delivery may be wise.

Interval Growth

In many clinical situations, it is impossible to confidently discriminate IUGR from a normal fetus with flawed dates. The symmetrically grown fetus, with normal amniotic fluid, and normal biophysical behavior, may appear IUGR if clinical dating is in error or represent one of the several IUGR etiologies associated with symmetric growth. Careful biometry on one occasion may not lead to a sure diagnosis. In such a case, serial growth evaluations at no less than 2-week intervals might add power to the assessment. If the infant parallels the normal growth curve, and all biophysical observations remain reassuring, it is unlikely that uteroplacental insufficiency is present. Discrimination of symmetric IUGR from flawed dates might remain difficult, but, in the absence of uteroplacental insufficiency that would be indicated by further difference between observed and expected growth, the risk of fetal compromised is diminished. Fetal surveillance during the intervals between the serial growth assessments is recommended.

Although the symmetry and onset of growth delay relate to the etiology, neither aspect of a fetus by itself influences management. Management, once the diagnosis is made, is based on gestational age, velocity of growth, and fetal condition. Early, severe IUGR, on the other hand, raises the possibility of fetal aneuploidy, particularly trisomies 13 or 18, and fetal karyotype may be considered.

MACROSOMIA

Macrosomia may be defined as a birthweight over the 90th percentile for gestational age, birthweight over 4000 g in the diabetic patient, or birthweight over 4500 g in the nondiabetic. Macrosomia is of clinical significance not only because of a higher-than-average rate of cesarean delivery, but because of a relationship with birth trauma and shoulder dystocia. Although only half of all cases of shoulder dystocia occur in the macrosomic group, the relative risk of shoulder dystocia exceeds 20% as birthweight rises over 4500 g in the nondiabetic and over 4000 g in the diabetic. Therefore, several authors have suggested the possible utility of sonographic EFW in the perinatal management of the pregnancy with suspected macrosomia.

However, if the sonographic estimation of fetal weight is to be used as the basis for consideration of operative delivery, the precision of the technique becomes critical (Fig. 6-7A–D). Since the currently used methods all have an error range of about ±10% for a single standard deviation, 67% of the estimates will be within 10% of the actual birthweight. Half of the estimates will be greater than the actual birthweight, and half will be less. In clinical decision making, we are most interested in the probability that the actual birthweight will be at least above a given diagnostic level, be it 4000 g or 4500 g. In order to be sure at a confidence level of 80% that the birthweight is at least 4000 g, the estimate would have to be over 4400 g. For a similar level of confidence at 4500 g, the estimate would have to be over 5400 g.

The logical conclusion is that sonographic estimation of fetal weight is only one of several variables to be taken into account when considering cesarean delivery to avoid shoulder dystocia. The estimated fetal weight threshold for considering operative delivery in the case of the obese diabetic with an unfavorable pelvic examination may be lower than that for the appropriate weight nondiabetic with a favorable examination. The choice of delivery method in the case of prolonged second stage may be different in the case of an obese diabetic with an EFW of 4500 g when compared with a nondiabetic of average weight with an estimated fetal weight of 3800 g.

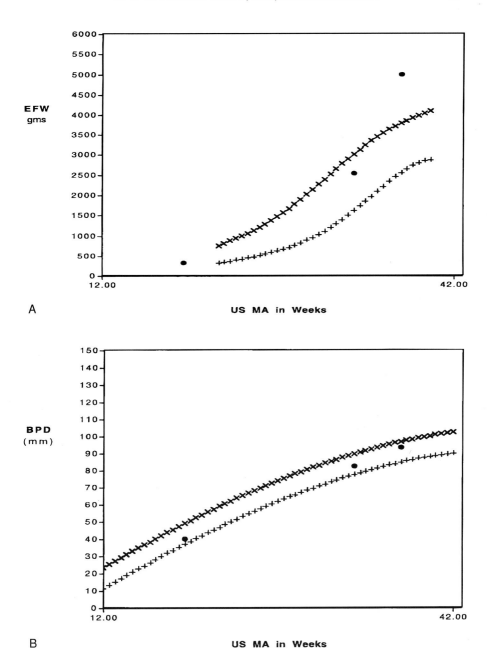

A

US MA in Weeks

B

US MA in Weeks

FIG. 6-7. A: Sequential EFW in the case of macrosomia shows the EFW clearly exceeding the 90th percentile only late in the third trimester. **B:** Sequential BPD tracking, however, shows this measure remaining within normal limits.

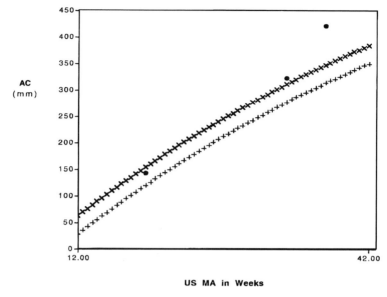

C

US MA in Weeks

D

US MA in Weeks

FIG. 6-7 *(Continued.)* **C:** The AC, as in the case of IUGR, clearly shows unique excessive growth in the case of macrosomia. **D:** The FL may be the only fetal dimension accurately reflecting fetal gestational age, as it remains within the normal range even in this fetus with very augmented growth.

FURTHER READING

Acker DB, Gregory KD, Sachs BP, *et al*. Risk factors for Erb-Duchene palsy. *Obstet Gynecol* 1988;71:389.

Acker DB, Sachs BP, Friedman EA. Risk factors for shoulder dystocia. *Obstet Gynecol* 1985;66:762.

Boyd ME, Usher RH, McLean FH. Fetal macrosomia prediction, risks, and proposed management. *Obstet Gynecol* 1983;61:715.

Bracero LA, Baxi LV, Rey HR, Yeh MN. Use of ultrasound in antenatal diagnosis of large for gestational age infants in diabetic gravid patients. *Am J Obstet Gynecol* 1985;152:43.

Gross SJ, Shime J, Farine D. Shoulder dystocia: predictors and outcome. *Am J Obstet Gynecol* 1987;156:334.

Ott WJ. Clinical application of fetal weight determination by realtime ultrasound measurements. *Obstet Gynecol* 1981;57:758.

Ott WJ, Doyle S. Ultrasonic diagnosis of altered fetal growth by use of a normal ultrasonic fetal weight curve. *Obstet Gynecol* 1984;63:201.

Rose BI, McCallum WD. A simplified method for estimating fetal weight using ultrasound measurements. *Obstet Gynecol* 1987;69:671.

Seeds JW. Impaired fetal growth: ultrasonic evaluation and clinical management. *Obstet Gynecol* 1984;64:577.

Shepard MJ, Richards VA, Berkowitz RL, *et al*. An evaluation of two equations for predicting fetal weight by ultrasound. *Am J Obstet Gynecol* 1982;142:47.

Warsoff SL, Gohari P, Berkowitz RL, *et al*. The estimation of fetal weight by computer assisted analysis. *Am J Obstet Gynecol* 1977;129:881.

Weinberger E, Cyr DR, Hirsch JH, *et al*. Estimating fetal weights less than 2000 g: an accurate and simple method. *AJR* 1984;141:973.

Woo JSK, Wan MCW. An evaluation of fetal weight prediction using a simple equation containing the fetal femur length. *J Ultrasound Med* 1986;5:453.

Yarkoni S, Reece EA, Wan M, *et al*. Intrapartum fetal weight estimation: a comparison of three formulae. *J Ultrasound Med* 1986;5:707.

7

Ultrasound and the Assessment of Fetal Condition

The antenatal evaluation of fetal well-being has been traditionally based on the accumulation of a variety of data that are indirectly reflective of fetal condition including

1. Adequacy of fetal growth
2. Fetal heart rate patterns
    unstressed reactivity
    response to contractions
3. Maternally monitored daily fetal movements
4. Sonographic biophysical profile
5. Doppler velocimetry

In addition, direct evidence of fetal condition is available using fetal blood sampling to assess fetal oxygenation and acid-base balance, both in the antepartum and intrapartum period. Percutaneous fetal blood sampling allows fetal blood gas analysis in the antepartum period, while scalp blood sampling is a well-established method for assessment of fetal scalp blood pH in the intrapartum situation.

Investigational techniques for the assessment of fetal well-being include Doppler evaluation of fetal arterial blood velocity patterns as well as fetal pulse oximetry.

Any system of periodic surveillance is based on the thesis that deterioration of the intrauterine environment and fetal condition is a gradual process. In the majority of cases this is true, but cord accidents, placental abruption, and rupture of membranes with cord prolapse cannot be predicted or prevented. Therefore, despite the appropriate use of any method of fetal surveillance, fetal deaths will occur at a rate of about 1–2/1000.

After a brief review of nonsonographic methodology, we will explore sonographic methods including biophysical profile testing (BPP), and Doppler velocimetry.

ELECTRONIC FETAL HEART RATE TESTING

The fetal heart beats with an intrinsic rhythm established by the sinoatrial node. This intrinsic rhythmicity is modulated by the autonomic nervous system. Parasympathetic (vagal) discharge slows the heart, and sympathetic discharge (catecholamine) increases the rate. The basic parameters of the fetal heart rate that are important are the **baseline rate** (normal 120–160), **reactivity** (accelerations from sympathetic discharge typically after fetal movement), **beat-to-beat variability** (parasympathetic discharge), and the presence or absence of **periodic decelerations** (early, late, or variable). Late decelerations have been associated with fetal hypoxemia, and loss of beat-to-beat variability of the baseline has been associated with fetal acidosis. Late decelerations begin after the contraction, drop slowly to a nadir near the end of the contraction, and return to baseline slowly after the contraction.

The earliest methods of antepartum fetal surveillance assessed fetal heart rate during maternal physical exercise. Decelerations during maternal exertion were thought to indicate a lack of uteroplacental respiratory reserve and the need for delivery. More recently, the stress applied to detect placental insufficiency is uterine contractions. Contractions occurring spontaneously, or because of dilute pitocin or nipple stimulation at a required rate of three per 10-minute period produce the stress, and fetal condition is inferred from heart rate responses. Late decelerations in response to at least two out of three uterine contractions indicate the possibility of fetal compromise. The most accurate prediction of fetal compromise is the combination of a nonreactive positive contraction stress test. Nonstressed fetal heart rate testing evolved empirically from the observation that, in most cases, no late decelerations were seen when baseline accelerations were seen with fetal movements. Two accelerations of at least 15 beats per minute for 15 seconds in a 20-minute interval indicate functional competence of the autonomic nervous system.

CONTRACTION STRESS TEST (CST)

The observation of late decelerations with two out of three contractions occurring at a minimum rate of three contractions of palpable strength per 10 minutes either spontaneously, as a result of nipple stimulation, or as a result of dilute pitocin infusion constitutes a positive contraction stress test. Absence of decelerations is a negative test and, if clinically indicated, should be repeated in 1 week. A positive test indicates that induction of labor should be considered. Up to 50% of fetuses with a positive CST will, however, successfully tolerate induction of labor and vaginal delivery.

NONSTRESS TEST (NST)

The observation during fetal heart rate monitoring in the absence of contractions of two accelerations of 15 beats per minute lasting 15 seconds associated with fetal movement during a 20-minute period constitutes a normal reactive result. The test should be repeated in 1 week or sooner if clinical events indicate. If accelerations are not noted, the observation period may be extended to 40 minutes or repeated later in the day. Up to 20% of high-risk patients will have a nonreactive NST during the antenatal period. Fewer than 10% of these infants are truly compromised. Therefore, the appropriate next step is either a biophysical profile or a contraction stress test. If spontaneous decelerations are noted, further testing is indicated that should include ultrasound since severe oligohydramnios is often associated with such decelerations, and delivery might be indicated.

The nonstress test assesses the functional competence of the fetal central nervous system at the time and under the specific circumstances of testing. Such an assessment cannot predict the level of respiratory reserve of the placenta if circumstances change. If uterine activity increases or maternal uteroplacental perfusion deteriorates at some later time, the nonstress test cannot perfectly predict the fetal response. The contraction stress test, on the other hand, in measuring the fetal response to a given stress, is more reflective of fetal reserve and would retain some predictive value even if uterine activity increases or maternal condition deteriorates. The contraction stress test is viewed by many observers, therefore, as the more sensitive of the two tests, but by far the more expensive and cumbersome.

BIOPHYSICAL PROFILE

Another clinical method for monitoring fetal condition is the sonographic biophysical profile (BPP). The observation over two decades ago that, if fetal breathing movements are seen both meconium and fetal deaths are less frequent, initiated interest in these observations. The relationship between amniotic fluid volume and fetal urine output led to interest in this parameter of well-being. The basis of a relationship between fetal urine output and well-being is found in the typical fetal response to stress that includes a redistribution of fetal cardiac output favoring brain, adrenals, and coronary arteries at the expense of other organs, especially kidneys. Therefore, oligohydramnios is associated with chronic fetal stress.

In 1979, Manning and Platt reported the combination of NST, breathing movements, trunk movements, tone (limb movements), and amniotic fluid volume as the biophysical profile. Since that time, investigators have suggested that breathing movements are perhaps the first lost and the most sensitive for marginal fetal status, and that absence of gross body movements is the most predictive of impending fetal demise. Fetal breathing movements represent lowering of the diaphragm (Fig. 7-1), with contraction of the fetal chest and expansion of the fetal abdomen (Fig. 7-2) in a rhythmic movement.

Using realtime ultrasound, the fetus is examined for fetal breathing movements (Fig. 7-3), trunk and limb movements, and the volume of amniotic fluid is evaluated. These observations are combined with the results of the nonstress test to provide a score of 0 to 10. The initial report used a single amniotic fluid pocket

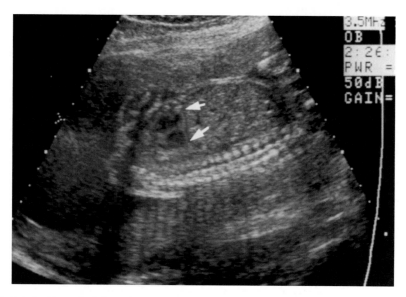

FIG. 7-1. In this sagittal view of a fetus, the diaphragm may be seen *(arrows)*. Contraction of the diaphragm and apparent "breathing movements" may be detected as early as 15 weeks and appear to indicate an intact and functional brainstem.

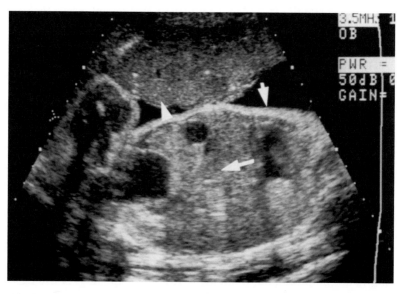

FIG. 7-2. As indicated here, breathing movements involve the contraction of the diaphragm *(large arrow),* contraction of the chest *(short arrow),* and expansion of the abdomen *(arrowhead).*

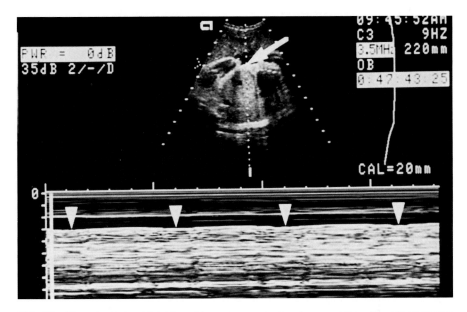

FIG. 7-3. M-mode study of fetal breathing movements can document this dynamic phenomenon. Note the M-mode cursor passing through the fetal chest just above the diaphragm. Note also below, the contraction of the chest *(arrowheads)* with each breathing movement.

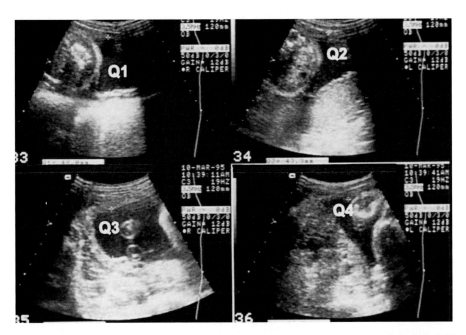

FIG. 7-4. The amniotic fluid index (AFI) is derived of the greatest vertical pocket of amniotic fluid not including cord, within each of the four frontal quadrants of the uterus. Illustrated here are the four measurements. The cord may be within the scanplane but should not be included in the measurement.

TABLE 7–1. *Biophysical profile scoring*

Observation	Score
Breathing movements	2 (30 seconds/30 minutes)
Trunk movements	2 (3 in 30 minutes)
Limb flex/ext	2 (3 in 30 minutes)
Amniotic fluid volume	2 (AFI over 5)
Reactive nonstress test	2

of 1 cm diameter as a threshold for awarding two points for amniotic fluid or not, but most observers agree that 1 cm is too severe, and the threshold was increased to 2 cm. More recently, the substitution of the amniotic fluid index (AFI) of 5 cm or less has been widely adopted. The AFI is the aggregate of the greatest vertical measure of amniotic fluid in each of the four frontal quadrants of the uterus (Fig. 7-4).

BIOPHYSICAL PROFILE SCORING

A BPP score of 8–10 is normal, 4–6 is questionable, and, repeated in 24 hours, 0–2 indicates the need for immediate delivery (see Table 7-1). Most observers have noted that each of the parameters, if normal, is equally predictive of a fetus in good condition, but that the whole BPP, if the score is low, is the best predictor of a compromised fetus. A poor BPP is a better predictor of fetal distress than a nonreactive NST, but a normal BPP is no better than a reactive NST. Furthermore, although a 30-minute observation period is required to score a zero for movement parameters, on average, only 8–10 minutes is required for a BPP, since the majority of fetuses are in good condition and will provide the needed information quickly.

Attempts to modify the BPP with intermediate scores of 1 for intermediate observations, resulting in aggregate totals of 1, 3, 5, 7, 9 for the BPP or adding placental grading as a sixth element with a maximum score possible of 12, have been reported without convincing evidence of superior performance. Modified BPP systems have not become standard. As mentioned before, some have suggested that fetal breathing movements were the most sensitive indicator of brain hypoxia, while others appear to show that absent fetal movements are the most predictive of proximate fetal death.

IMPACT OF CIRCUMSTANCES

Biophysical scoring, as with other forms of passive indirect fetal monitoring, are **circumstance dependent.** The condition of the fetus at the moment of testing under the exact conditions of testing is being evaluated. The predictive value for fetal survival for a given period of time depends on the constancy of those circumstances. Increased maternal blood pressure, fever, increased uterine tonus or activity, are all circumstances that might alter fetal condition and, therefore, the predictive value of any recent passive monitoring method loses its value. We cannot guarantee a fetus with a normal NST or BPP. We can reassure the patient that, given normal results and constant circumstances, the perinatal mortality within a week of a normal test is not zero, but very low, about 1–2/1000. The patient needs to be informed that prolonged unmonitored labor is not necessarily safe simply because of a recent reassuring test result.

The observation during an obstetric ultrasound of fetal activity such as breathing, trunk, or limb movements, is potentially valuable clinical information and should be noted in the report.

DOPPLER EVALUATION: DOPPLER EFFECT

Sound reflected from a moving object is altered in wavelength and frequency (see Chapter 1). If the object is moving toward the sound source, the wavelength of the echo is shorter and the frequency higher than the original sound, thus producing a positive Doppler effect or frequency shift. If the object is moving away from the source, the wavelength of the echo is longer and the frequency lower than the original, producing a negative Doppler effect, or frequency shift (see Figures in Chapter 1). The shift in frequency is proportional to the velocity of movement and is maximal if the direction of movement is exactly parallel to the direction of propagation of the sound pulses, called zero angle. If the direction of movement is at 90 degrees to the direction of propagation of the primary sound pulse, there is no change in frequency.

Continuous Wave Doppler

Fetal monitors, office Dopplers, and some available Doppler umbilical artery devices generate ultrasound energy continuously at low amplitude, and receive and analyze echoes continuously. These are low power, usually 6 mw/cm^2, and intermediate frequency, usually 4 megahertz. The Doppler frequency shifts are continuously displayed on a monitor by a computerized spectrum analyzer, giving a velocity profile that includes the maximum frequency shifts (maximum velocities) as well as intermediate values. Continuous wave (CW) equipment does not discriminate differential depths for echo signals nor is CW Doppler compatible with simultaneous imaging. Range gating is not possible, incorporation into imaging systems is not possible, therefore, there are severe limitations on the clinical usefulness of these systems. The operator cannot know precisely which vessel is being interrogated, or at what angle, and any movement of any object in the field will create noise. Patterns of frequency shift, however, may be evaluated and may be useful.

Duplex Doppler

The analysis of Doppler shift of reflected echoes in a pulse-echo system allows incorporation of the methodology into imaging systems, producing a duplex Doppler system. Such systems allow visualization of the vessel being interrogated, estimation of the angle of insonation, and, therefore, estimation of the actual velocity of movement (Fig. 7-5). Such systems are substantially more expensive than continuous wave systems, but they provide more information.

The Doppler effect can be quantitative or qualitative. The precise relationship between the frequency shift and the velocity of the moving object is

$$FreqShift = -2V \times Cos\ \theta \times FreqTrans \div 1540$$

or

$$Velocity = FreqShift \times 1540 \div Cos\ \theta \times FreqTrans \times 2$$

If the angle of insonation (interrogation, or the angle between the direction of the soundbeam and the direction of motion of the object) is known, therefore, the precise velocity of the object may be calculated. If the object is a blood cell in an artery, the volume flow might be estimated using the Doppler-derived velocity if

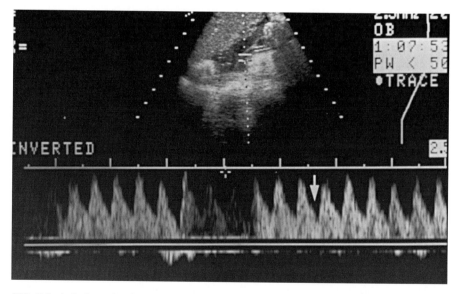

FIG. 7-5. A duplex pulse Doppler study of an umbilical artery in a normal pregnancy. Note the pulsatility of the signal, the systolic peak Doppler shift (proportional to velocity not necessarily volume flow), and the diastolic nadir *(arrow)*. The ratio of the systolic peak to the diastolic nadir (S/D) has been used to follow gestation but has not shown superior performance to traditional monitoring methods.

the cross-sectional area of the vessel were known. Useful interrogation sites include the umbilical artery, the umbilical vein, the middle cerebral artery, the ductus arteriosus, and the thoracic aorta. However, volume flow has not proved to be a useful parameter since the area of a pulsatile arterial vessel is in constant flux, and the velocity of red cells is not constant across the vessel.

Doppler Parameters

The evaluation of the Doppler waveform (Fig. 7-5) is typically based on the ratio of systolic peak to diastolic nadir frequency shift in the arterial signal, on the presence or absence of the umbilical artery (UA) diastolic flow, or on the presence of periodic umbilical veinous velocity pulsations.

Clinical Utility

Early investigators attempted to use Doppler to measure blood flow. However, imprecise determination of vessel size and angle of insonation renders these efforts variable and inaccurate. Furthermore, the variable corpuscular flow in a blood vessel makes no one velocity an accurate measure of flow. Therefore, recent efforts have concentrated on largely qualitative evaluation of the shape or profile of velocities or frequency shifts from a vessel. The comparison of systolic maximum (S) to diastolic minimum (D) is considered proportional to downstream impedance and, therefore, perhaps reflective of either a pathologic vascular bed or a vasospastic bed.

The S/D ratio has been used as a qualitative measure of resistance (impedance). It is not necessary to know or to standardize the angle of insonation to calculate the S/D ratio. However, near zero angle insonation is best, since low-velocity diastolic flow may be lost in the noise if insonation near 90 degrees is attempted. The vessel diameter is likewise not relevant. Another measure of impedance is the Pulsatility Index, which is S-D/Mean. Both have been used in clinical trials. In the case of absent diastolic flow, the S/D ratio becomes useless, however, while the pulsatility index remains useful.

The S/D ratio of the umbilical artery shows a high diastolic velocity that increases with gestational age in the normal fetus. The S/D ratio has been shown to decline from 2.8 to 2.2 between 25 and 41 weeks gestation. An S/D ratio over 3.0 has been associated with IUGR, but, as a diagnostic tool, sensitivity and specificity have been disappointing. A rising S/D ratio has been associated with deteriorating fetal condition. Absence of diastolic flow is seen in the highest risk situations but does not appear to be an acutely reactive event. In other words, absent diastolic flow, as a measure of the pathology of small villus vessels, does not evolve quickly or improve quickly if at all. But, the observation of absent end-diastolic flow (AEDF) in the context of other high-risk circumstances such as IUGR or pregnancy-induced hypertension identifies a fetus at substantially higher risk than the fetus with good diastolic flow on the basis that one villus circulation is healthier than the other.

Randomized clinical trials evaluating Doppler velocimetry as a basis for management have shown eqivocal differences in outcome. Therefore, although Doppler-derived umbilical-artery S/D ratio or pulsatility or resistance indices add additional insight into the pathophysiology of the fetus, it is premature to conclude that this new approach is better than the more traditional methods for the assessment of fetal condition.

Trudinger, in 1987, reported a study of 300 high-risk patients who underwent Doppler umbilical artery surveillance antenatally, with the results reported in half of the cases and not reported in the others. The results showed no substantial difference in perinatal outcome. Newnham, in 1991, reported a similar study of 545 patients with 275 in the Doppler group and 270 in the control group, and again there was no significant difference in clinical outcome. Johnstone, in 1993, reported a randomized trial from Glasgow that included over 2200 patients, with no significant difference in outcome with the use of Doppler surveillance techniques. Routine use of Doppler velocimetry for surveillance of high-risk pregnancies, therefore, is not an accepted standard.

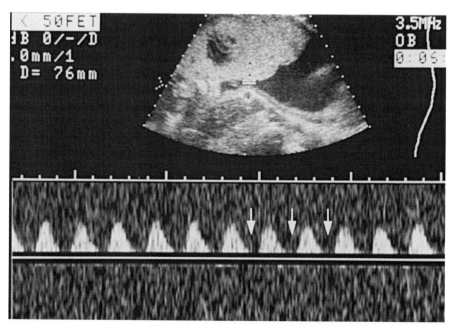

FIG. 7-6. Absence of end-diastolic flow (absence of diastolic Doppler shift indicated by *arrows*) is an ominous finding. The highest perinatal risk is associated with this type of pattern, and careful perinatal surveillance and attention is indicated. A decrease in venous velocity coincident with the AEDF is even more ominous.

Investigational uses that compare waveforms of the umbilical artery to those of the fetal cerebral vessels may identify those fetuses with the "brain sparing" effect of blood flow redistribution that has characterized deprivational circumstances, but the clinical value remains unproved. Asymmetry of growth is another reflection of the altered distribution of cardiac output in the chronically stressed fetus.

Absent End-Diastolic Flow and Venous Pulsations

Absent end-diastolic flow (Fig. 7-6) has been observed by many to identify the most compromised fetus. Although randomized clinical trials have not shown that Doppler studies in general result overall in better salvage than traditional monitoring techniques, most investigators agree that loss of end-diastolic flow may be seen prior to other indicators of impending fetal compromise. Investigators have found a high rate of cesarean deliveries, perinatal mortality, and anomalies associated with loss of fetal umbilical artery diastolic flow.

Decreased umbilical venous velocity (venous pulsations) coinciding with absent end-diastolic flow indicates a failing right ventricle and may even be associated with reverse fetal inferior vena caval flow and tricuspid regurgitation. These venous "pulsations" appear to represent a peripheral reflection of extreme fetal compromise and identify the fetus that requires delivery. Venous pulsations associated with absent end-diastolic flow appear to be the endstage signs of fetal cardiovascular failure.

OTHER NEW MODALITIES

Techniques have been reported for the use of continuous fetal scalp pH monitoring and continuous fetal scalp pO_2 monitoring using special glass electrodes. Although continuous monitoring might offer some theoretical advantages over intermittent sampling, such devices are not likely to become widely available due to difficulties in miniaturization of the fiberoptic light delivery and light detection apparatus. It is unlikely that such infrared light absorption will be able to measure fetal brain oxygen in an absolute fashion but rather will provide relative oxygenation information from which patterns may be recognized that indicate fetal well-being or fetal distress. Such technical adaption and clinical evaluation will likely require considerable time.

Fetal pulse oximetry during the intrapartum period is possible and is under clinical investigation.

CONCLUSIONS

Under constant clinical circumstances, nonstress fetal testing is adequate primary surveillance. If circumstances change, increased frequency of NST or contraction stress testing appears to be more sensitive to uteroplacental respiratory reserve capacity. In the case of a nonreactive NST, either a biophysical profile or a contraction stress test are useful backup tests. The full biophysical profile is the best predictor of a compromised fetus when abnormal. None of the current methods can perfectly anticipate or prevent fetal death. Doppler arterial waveform analysis offers some additional insight but no confirmed clinical advantages over conventional methods, but absent end-diastolic flow, if observed (especially if accompanied by venous pulsations), indicates serious uteroplacental deficiency.

FURTHER READING

Baskett TF, *et al.* Fetal biophysical profile and perinatal death. *Obstet Gynecol* 1987;70:357.

Baskett TF, Gray JH, Prewett SJ, Young LM, Allen AC. Antepartum fetal assessment using a fetal biophysical profile score. *Am J Obstet Gynecol* 1984;148:(5)630–3.

Baskett TF, Sandy EA. The oxytocin challenge test: an ominous pattern associated with severe fetal growth retardation. *Obstet & Gynecol.* 1979;54(3):365–6.

Evertson LR, *et al.* Antepartum fetal heart rate testing. I. Evolution of the nonstress test. *Am J Obstet Gynecol* 1979;133:29.

Freeman RK. The use of the oxytocin challenge test for antepartum clinical evaluation of uteroplacental respiratory function. *Am J Obstet Gynecol* 1975;121(4):481–9.

Johnstone FD, Prescott R, Hoskins P, *et al.* The effect of introduction of umbilical Doppler recordings to obstetric practice. *Br J Obstet Gynaecol* 1993;100:733–41.

Low JA. The current status of maternal and fetal blood flow velocimetry. *Am J Obstet Gynecol* 1991;164: 1049–63.

Manning FA, Harman CR, Morrison I, Menticoglou SM, *et al.* Fetal assessment based on fetal biophysical profile scoring. IV. An analysis of perinatal morbidity and mortality. *Am J Obstet Gynecol* 1990; 162:703–9.

Mandruzzato GP, Bogatti P, Fischer L, Gigli C. The clinical significance of absent or reverse end-diastolic flow in the fetal aorta and umbilical artery. *Ultrasound Obstet Gynecol* 1991;1:192–6.

Mari G, Moise KJ, Deter RL, *et al.* Doppler assessment of the pulsatility index in the cerebral circulation of the human fetus. *Am J Obstet Gynecol* 1989;160:698–703.

Newnham JP, O'Dea MR, Reid KP, Diepeveen DA. Doppler flow velocity waveform analysis in high risk pregnancies: a randomized controlled trial. *Br J Obstet Gynaecol* 1991;98:956–63.

Pattinson RC, Norman K, Odendaal HJ: The role of Doppler velocimetry in the management of high risk pregnancies. *Br J Obstet Gynaecol* 1994;101:114–20.

Phalen JP, Cromartie AD, Smith CV. The nonstress test: the false negative test. *Am J Obstet Gynecol* 1982; 142:293.

Rochelson B, Schulman H, Farmakides G, *et al.* The significance of absent end-diastolic velocity in umbilical artery velocity waveforms. *Am J Obstet Gynecol* 1987;156:1213–8.

Schulman H. *et al.* Umbilical velocity wave ratios in human pregnancy. *Am J Obstet Gynecol* 1984;148: 985.

Trudinger BJ, Cook CM. Umbilical and uterine artery flow velocity waveforms in pregnancy associated with major fetal abnormality. *Br J Obstet Gynecol* 1985;92:666.

Trudinger BJ, Giles WB, Cook CM. Flow velocity waveforms in the maternal uteroplacental and fetal umbilical placental circulations. *Am J Obstet Gynecol* 1985;152:155.

Vintzileos AM, *et al.* The relationship between fetal biophysical profile and cord pH in patients undergoing cesarean section before the onset of labor. *Obstet Gynecol* 1987;70:196.

Vyas S, Nicolaides KH, Bower S, Campbell S. Middle cerebral artery flow velocity waveforms in fetal hypoxaemia. *Br J Obstet Gynaecol* 1990;97:797–803.

8

Complementary Obstetric Applications

This chapter addresses the methodology of ultrasound direction of intracorporeal procedures and fetal manipulation. The technical options available to the practitioner are described.

INVASIVE OBSTETRIC PROCEDURES

Amniocentesis

Amniocentesis is readily directed by transabdominal realtime ultrasound techniques. Guidance may be accomplished utilizing linear, sector, or curvilinear transducers. The sector or curvilinear transducers offer more versatility and allow detection of the needle tip earlier in the procedure while the needle tip is still in the subcutaneous tissue. For these reasons most operators favor either the sector or curvilinear transducer for direction of transabdominal procedures.

The technique of needle guidance can be performed utilizing the plane of the scanning beam (co-planar) or utilizing a plane perpendicular to the scanning beam (trans-planar). The co-planar (parallel) technique allows visualization of the length of the needle whereas the transplanar technique allows visualization of the echo generated by the scanning beam intersecting the needle. The latter technique mandates frequent back and forth movement of the transducer to assure that the tip of the needle is being visualized (Figs. 8-1,8-2).

The technique begins with selection of the most favorable amniocentesis site. Scanning perpendicular to the uterine surface (in contrast to the plane of the exam table) will allow selection of an area (pocket) of amniotic fluid to be sampled. Ideally, one would prefer not to traverse the placenta and, also, to avoid the fetal head and body. If a transplacental approach is necessary, the umbilical cord insertion site should be avoided.

After the sampling site is selected, the abdomen is prepared with antiseptic solution and, depending upon patient desire and physician preference, local anes-

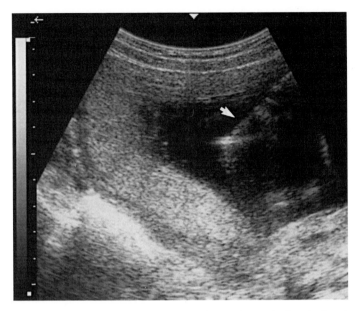

FIG. 8-1. Orientation of the transducer in a co-planar image format depicts the length of the amniocentesis needle within the amniotic sac *(arrow)*. Note the bright echo of the needle tip.

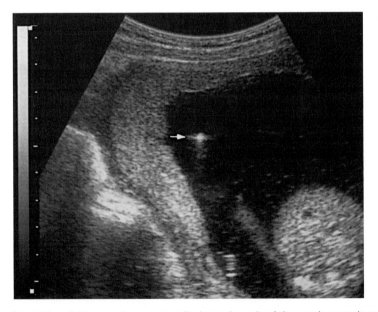

FIG. 8-2. Orientation of the transducer perpendicular to the axis of the amniocentesis needle (trans-planar) results in visualization of the needle where the scanning beam transects the shaft *(arrow)*. Utilizing this approach, one must continually adjust the scanning plane to assure that the tip of the needle is being imaged and not a cross-sectional portion of the needle shaft.

thesia (approximately 1 cc lidocaine without epinephrine) is placed in the subcutaneous tissue. Many operators do not use local anesthesia due to the minimal discomfort of the cutaneous component of the needle passage and the discomfort of the anesthetic solution. Others favor the use of lidocaine to promote patient relaxation and, cooperation, and to minimize anxiety.

Many options exist to avoid contamination of the sterile field by the transducer. Most operators utilize some form of transducer sheathing with a sterile synthetic transducer cover. Any technique to prevent contamination of the field is acceptable. Sterilized sandwich bags or commercially available transducer covers both suffice for this purpose. A freehand technique that merely avoids the insertion site is also feasible but mandates constant awareness of the relationship of the transducer and the sterile field.

If the co-planar technique is utilized, the transducer is positioned in a parallel plane to the axis of the needle (18–22 g), and the needle-tip echo is sought in the subcutaneous tissue. At this point, the operator should concentrate on keeping the needle essentially perpendicular to the abdominal wall (since this was the orientation of the transducer that was utilized to select the area to be sampled) and should avoid the tendency to angle the needle to a more tangential plane under the transducer in an effort to enhance its visualization. If tangential deflection of the needle occurs, the myometrium will be entered in a tangential plane producing more patient discomfort, difficulty in accessing the preselected sampling site, and necessitating unnecessary needle manipulation.

The needle, once visualized, should be directed in a steady, smooth manner into the preselected area of amniotic fluid. If there is concern about fetal puncture, the operator should cease the insertion, await spontaneous fetal movement out of the area, and/or redirect the needle into a more favorable area.

The physician may use a freehand technique or use an attachable biopsy guide. The latter approach provides a visible insertion path seen on the monitor but also mandates less maneuverability for possible redirection needed by fetal movement. With experience, most operators prefer the freehand technique for amniocentesis.

If an amniocentesis is being performed relatively early in the second trimester, a quicker and abbreviated puncture of the amnion may be required to avoid separating the amnion from the underlying chorion and tenting of the amnion. If this does occur, the operator must attempt to puncture the amnion in the same plane or locate an alternative site and begin the process again.

Ultrasound guidance of the needle may be performed by an assistant or the operator. Visualization of the needle tip throughout the aspiration of amniotic fluid will assist in any necessary manipulation of the needle tip. In addition, the patient may be reassured that no fetal trauma is occurring if she can visualize the needle tip throughout the procedure.

Following removal of the needle, the insertion site is visualized for any evidence of bleeding and the fetal status is again confirmed. A post-procedure segment of videotape is suggested to document fetal status and lack of bleeding at the amniocentesis site.

If an amniocentesis is being performed on multiple sacs, the operator may use a single puncture technique in which more than one sac is entered by redirecting the needle. An alternative, and more widely used technique, is to use separate needle insertions for each sac in order to avoid creating defects in the membranes between the sacs. These defects may increase in size and potentially allow cord or fetal entanglement to occur.

If separate percutaneous sites are utilized, the instillation of 1–2 cc of indigo carmine as a marker for the first sac will assure that separate sacs have been sampled. Methylene blue should not be used for this purpose.

Regardless of which technique is elected, careful attention must be paid to the location of the amniotic sacs, orientation of the fetus, and the placentation site. Each sample must be labeled in a manner that will assure the correlation of the amniotic fluid results and the amniotic sac sampled. Sketches of fetal orientation and membrane status are helpful in this regard.

Percutaneous Umbilical (Fetal) Blood Sampling

Fetal blood may safely be sampled by percutaneous aspiration of fetal blood from the umbilical vessels (preferably umbilical vein) utilizing ultrasound guidance. The technique for ultrasound-directed fetal blood sampling is similar to the procedure of guided amniocentesis.

In the cordocentesis procedure, the umbilical vein is accessed using a 20–22 g needle under continuous ultrasound direction. The umbilical cord is most easily entered at a site of relative immobility such as the umbilical insertion of the fetus, or, more frequently, the insertion of the umbilical cord into the placenta. The placental insertion site may be entered either perpendicularly to the vessel wall or from a direction parallel to the axis of the umbilical vein by traversing the placental stroma. If neither of these sites is accessible, a free loop of cord may be tried. The tendency for the free loop to float away from the sampling needle must be kept in mind.

As the needle tip approaches the vessel, one must be careful to fine-tune the orientation of the transducer scanning plane, the vessel wall, and the needle tip. Once the vessel wall is approximated utilizing the parallel (co-planar) technique, rotation of the transducer 90 degrees to visualize the axial plane (trans-planar orientation) of the vessel will allow the operator to position the needle tip in the mid-lumen of the umbilical vein.

Access to the umbilical vein allows phlebotomy for fetal hematologic study and the opportunity to infuse the fetus directly with medications and/or blood. Analogous to amniocentesis, this procedure mandates strict adherence to aseptic technique.

Complications of this procedure include transient bleeding from the aspiration site and fetal bradycardia. Because these complications occasionally result in the need for emergency delivery, this procedure should be performed in proximity to a delivery area where an emergency cesarean section may safely be performed.

Fetal Intracorporeal Aspiration and Shunting

Ultrasound guidance allows access to diagnostic and/or therapeutic centesis procedures at a variety of sites. Whether this involves aspirating fluid from the fetal thorax, pericardium, abdomen, or urinary tract, the procedure is essentially the same as described above.

The rationale, indications, contraindications, and complications of placing intracorporeal-amniotic shunts are all areas of current investigational interest. The technique is also analogous to that described above. The shunting catheter/cannula is threaded over a centesis needle and is pushed off of the needle into the desired location. In all likelihood, an ever-increasing body of literature will require continued reassessment to determine what role these techniques will eventually have in modern obstetric practice.

Chorionic Villi Sampling (CVS)

The aspiration of chorionic villi in the first trimester allows accurate karyotyping of the fetus by evaluating the chromosomal status of the trophoblastic villi. Trophoblastic villi may be obtained by either a transabdominal or transvaginal approach.

The transabdominal approach is performed in similar fashion to ultrasound-directed amniocentesis. In this procedure, the sampling needle is directed into the chorion frondosum. The ideal candidate for this approach is one with an anteverted uterus and the placenta implanted on the anterior uterine wall or in the uterine fundus. Chorionic villi are aspirated by applying negative pressure via a 20 cc syringe. Several passes of the needle may be necessary to obtain an adequate sample of villi. An adequate sample is approximately 5 mg or more.

To avoid the necessity of multiple insertions of the needle through the patient's skin, some operators prefer to insert a larger bore needle under ultrasound guidance into the proximal portion of the area to be sampled and pass a smaller gauge needle through the larger one as many times as needed to obtain an acceptable sample. This technique has been referred to as the *needle within a needle* technique.

Transvaginal approaches for villi sampling may be performed by a transcervical approach or a needle puncture of the upper vagina and the uterine wall. The latter technique is guided by an endovaginal transducer and involves a transvaginal insertion into the chorion frondosum. This approach, which is rarely indicated, has been suggested to allow sampling of a patient with a markedly retroverted uterus and a posterior wall implantation site. Concern over infection makes this technique somewhat controversial.

These placenta sites may be sampled via a transcervical technique with uterine manipulation if needed in the vast majority of cases. With modest to minimal bladder filling, many retroverted uteri can be manipulated into a more anteverted orientation during the procedure, allowing access to the implantation site.

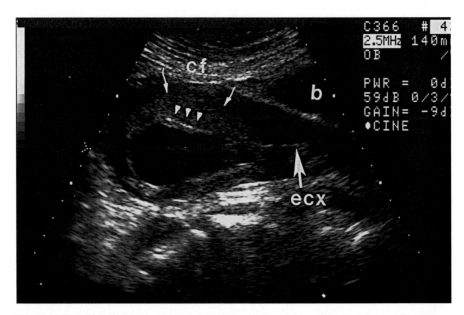

FIG. 8-3. The CVS catheter with stylet *(small arrowheads)* is within the chorion frondosum *(curved arrows* and marked *cf).* Note the sagittal image of the first-trimester uterus, endocervical canal *(ecx)* and maternal urinary bladder *(b).*

Virtually all vaginal CVS procedures are performed via the endocervical canal by inserting a small polyethylene catheter and directing it into the implantation site with continuous ultrasound guidance utilizing abdominal ultrasound performed by a skilled sonographer. The remainder of the technical description of this procedure will apply to the transcervical approach only (Fig. 8-3).

Following insertion of a bivalve speculum and appropriate application of antiseptic solution of the cervix, vagina, and lower genital tract, the sonographer and operator must decide upon the best approach to access the chorion frondosum. Ideally, the thickest area should be selected. The umbilical cord insertion site and yolk sac are important landmarks, but, utilizing modern high-resolution instrumentation, the selection of the thickest area is usually easily determined.

Some operators find it helpful to localize the endocervical os with a cotton-tipped applicator. This step will allow the sonographer to angle the transducer in a manner such that the desired sampling site and the internal cervical os are imaged in the same plane. By utilizing this method, the sonographer will more easily detect the catheter as soon as it enters the uterine cavity.

The sampling catheter is directed into the thickest area, and the stylet is removed. Aspiration pressure is applied via a 20 cc syringe, and the sampling catheter is slowly removed. Again a sample volume of >5 mg is desired. If an inadequate sample is achieved with the first attempt, a second attempt is acceptable. One must remember that the risk of an adverse outcome increases with more than two attempts to obtain villi. At the end of the procedure, a brief segment of videotape is suggested to confirm the status that exists at that time.

OTHER OBSTETRIC APPLICATIONS

Fetal Version

External version of the breech fetus allows avoidance of cesarean section in many patients. The resurgence of popularity of this technique can be attributed to four main modifications in the procedure in recent years. By avoiding maternal anesthesia, the likelihood of trauma from undue force is minimized. Secondly, the ability to monitor fetal heart rate allows detection of signs of cord entanglement. Thirdly, the use of tocolytics allows maximal uterine relaxation to enhance the success of the version. Lastly, and most important, transabdominal ultrasound allows the operator to define fetal position and monitor its attitude and orientation throughout the procedure.

Success rates of over 70% in properly selected patients have been reported. Determinants of success include the type of breech, placentation site, amniotic fluid volume, and parity. Breeches that are nonfrank breeches are more amenable to version. Anterior placentation, oligohydramnios, and primigravidity also decrease the likelihood of success.

An initial ultrasound will determine most of the important factors that influence the potential success or failure of the version. The vertex is located and the position of the fetal feet are noted. A forward-roll or back-flip technique is selected based upon which appears to be the most favorable. Using an abdominal lubricant (ultrasound couplant gel, for example) the fetus is gently rotated by one or both of the techniques mentioned above.

The procedure is best performed by slow, steady reorientation of the fetus with periodic assessment of fetal position and fetal heart rate. The latter may be performed by either ultrasound or fetal heart rate monitoring. Following manipulation, the fetal heart rate is monitored to detect any sign of cord vulnerability or entanglement by looking at heart rate, variability, and the presence or absence of period changes, especially variable or prolonged decelerations.

Due to the unlikely complications of abruptio placenta and/or cord entanglement, the procedure should be performed in an area with emergency cesarean section capability. In addition, appropriate staff should also be available. Lastly, the procedure should be performed late in the third trimester to minimize the risk of fetal prematurity and reversion to breech after successful version.

Management of the Second Nonvertex Twin

Abdominal ultrasound assessment of fetal position and attitude is also of benefit in the management of the nonvertex second twin. Location of the fetal feet for breech extraction or guiding version into a vertex presentation is aided by ultrasound. The delivery process can also be monitored using this technique.

Completion of Curettage

The completion of curettage of the endometrial cavity is possible by realtime ultrasound techniques. The transabdominal approach allows direct visualization of the procedure in progress. This technique is particularly useful in patients with uterine malposition, uterine anomaly, or those difficult to examine. The transvaginal approach allows detailed assessment of the uterine cavity following the procedure.

In the postpartum period, ultrasound offers assistance in directing the curette and avoiding uterine perforation. In addition, one can also be assured that all placental fragments have been removed.

SUMMARY

Realtime ultrasound offers the ability to direct a variety of obstetric procedures. The integration of this technology into the practice of obstetrics allows access to a great deal of important clinical information to assist the practitioner and benefit the maternal and fetal patients.

FURTHER READING

Benacerraf BR, Frigoletto FD. Amniocentesis under continuous ultrasound guidance: a series of 232 cases. *Obstet Gynecol* 1983;62:760–3.

Daffos F, Capella-Pavlovsky M, Forestier F. Fetal blood sampling during pregnancy with use of a needle guided by ultrasound: a study of 606 consecutive cases. *Am J Obstet Gynecol* 1985;153:655–60.

Elias S, Simpson JL, Shulman LP, Emerson D, Tharapel A, Seely L. Transabdominal chorionic villus sampling for first-trimester prenatal diagnosis. *Am J Obstet Gynecol* 1989;160:879–86.

Shulman LP, Simpson JL, Felker RE, Emerson DS, Meyer CM, Phillips OP, Elias S. Transvaginal chorionic villus sampling using transabdominal ultrasound guidance. *Prenat Diagn* 1992;12:229–34.

Wade RV, Young SR. Analysis of fetal loss after transcervical chorionic villus sampling—a review of 719 patients. *Am J Obstet Gynecol* 1989;161:513–9.

Wallace RL, VanDorsten JP, Eglinton GS, Mueller E, McCart D, Schifrin BS. External cephalic version with tocolysis. Observations and continuing experience at the Los Angeles County/University of Southern California Medical Center. *J Reprod Med* 1984;29:745–8.

9

The Role of Ultrasound in Maternal Serum Screening

Interest in sensitive and efficient antenatal screening of patients otherwise considered low risk for congenital disease in their fetuses has gained strength in the past two decades since the development of both maternal serum screening tests and high-resolution ultrasound. Historic screening early in prenatal care will identify certain patients at increased risk for a variety of reasons, including advanced maternal age and prior birth of an affected child. However, the large majority of congenital disease occurs in families with no prior history, and the majority of aneuploid fetuses are born to women under the age of 35. The earliest and simplest screening test was advanced maternal age. Although the age considered at risk has dropped over the years from 45 to 40 to 35, and in some areas even less, this gold standard risk indicator offers sensitivity of only 20% and a predictive value at age 35 of only 1/365 for liveborn Down syndrome at term. Furthermore, Down syndrome, indeed all aneuploidy, constitutes a small minority of the total of major congenital disease, and so, without mass screening techniques that focus on either broader populations or a larger variety of congenital defects, no great impact on the incidence of birth defects resulted.

Maternal serum alpha-fetoprotein (MSAFP) screening was the first such large-scale testing program that focused on the detection of a major malformation among otherwise low-risk patients. MSAFP screening originally focused only on the association of elevated MSAFP with open neural-tube defects but was quickly found to result in the detection of other malformations, including ventral wall defects and certain urinary tract anomalies that were all associated with severe oligohydramnios. In 1984, low levels of MSAFP were found to be associated with an increased risk of fetal trisomy. Maternal serum unconjugated estriol was later found to be similarly depressed in trisomy 21, and quantitative serum chorionic gonadotropin was found to be significantly elevated in patients with pregnancies complicated by fetal Down syndrome. The three markers together have been combined to form the "triple screen."

During this same period, investigators demonstrated the association between both major and minor fetal dysmorphology and aneuploidy. It is well known and not surprising that major fetal structural anomalies are associated with an increased rate of aneuploidy, but, in addition, over fifteen different minor dysmorphic features detectable by sonography have been examined and found to offer some value in screening for fetal aneuploidy.

Any study of this dynamic and emerging area of interest, therefore, must include an examination of the practical clinical value of both maternal serum screening and ultrasound in the evaluation of risk for fetal malformation.

MATERNAL SERUM ALPHA-FETOPROTEIN (MSAFP)

Alpha-fetoprotein (AFP) was first discovered in 1956 and was called "protein X." AFP is an important fetal serum protein made first in the yolk sac and later in the fetal liver and gut. Similar to albumin, and always exceeded in concentration by albumin, AFP peaks in fetal serum about 13–15 weeks' gestation and then falls precipitously. AFP concentration in amniotic fluid parallels this pattern at much lower levels. Although the physiologic purpose of AFP remains unclear, some speculate that AFP plays a role in inducing the immunologic privilege enjoyed by the fetal graft within the maternal host organism.

MSAFP, curiously, rises slowly to a peak at 32–34 weeks' gestation in ng/cc amounts in the normal pregnancy. The first observation of abnormal levels of AFP in the amniotic fluid of a fetus with anencephaly was reported in the early 1970s. Elevated MSAFP associated with other open neural tube defects was then subsequently reported, and the first pilot screening project was reported from England in 1974. The Scarborough Conference (held in Scarborough, Maine, 1977) examined the results of the British Collaborative Study and concluded that, although open neural tube defects occurred in much lower numbers in the USA (1-2/1000) than in England (4/1000), pilot screening projects were justified. U.S. pilot screening projects generally found similar diagnostic sensitivities to those expected from the English experience and, in 1985, the ACOG Department of Professional Liability concluded that MSAFP screening had reached a level of standard that each obstetric patient should be offered testing.

Fetal open neural tube defects (ONTD's) complicate 1–2/1000 pregnancies in the USA. The rate decreases from east to west. Alphafetoprotein is increased in the presence of fetal **ONTDs, ventral wall defects,** and **urinary tract defects** that produce anhydramnios.

MSAFP rises with gestational age, fetal death, and multiple gestation, therefore ultrasound may complement MSAFP screening at the simplest level by the confirmation of gestational age, fetal viability, and fetal number. This very basic type of sonographic examination was termed Level I by the Scarborough Conference. Ultrasound may also be used to search (Level II) specifically for the birth defects in question, but the training and experience necessary for optimal diagnostic sensitivity are not universal. A Level I ultrasound evaluation of patients with elevated MSAFP levels typically explains about **one third** on the basis of **dates, twins,** or **fetal death** (Table 9-1).

If MSAFP elevation is not explained by ultrasound, amniocentesis for assessment of amniotic fluid AFP is typically considered. The discovery of elevated amniotic fluid AFP and the detection of amniotic fluid acetylcholinesterase would confirm the presence of an open neural tube defect. However, amniocentesis carries risks, and the benefits must be weighed against these risks. The benefit of amniocentesis in the case of elevated MSAFP but a normal ultrasound is the possible detection of unseen ONTDs. The main risk of amniocentesis is pregnancy loss, often quoted as 0.5%, or 1/200. The sensitivity of ultrasound for the detection of ONTDs must be considered, because if an ultrasound examination performed by someone skilled and experienced in the detection of ONTDs fails to detect any evidence of a defect, the patient's risk is naturally less than that expected on the basis of MSAFP alone.

Clearly, a diagnostic sensitivity of 100% is expected in the case of anencephaly, and anencephaly constitutes about half of all ONTDs. Direct sonographic detection of spina bifida, however, was historically reported to provide only 50–80% sensitivity. On the basis of these considerations, many screening programs have not adjusted patient-specific neural tube defect risk from MSAFP because of a normal ultrasound examination.

In recent years, however, the observation of cranial and intracranial anatomic changes associated with ONTDs has greatly enhanced the ability of ultrasound to detect spina bifida. Five cranial features associated with spina bifida have been described, including a **biparietal diameter small** for dates, frontoparietal **indentation** or **notching** on the occipitofrontal scanplane (lemon sign), mild **ventriculomegaly, cerebellar compression deformity** (banana sign), and **obliteration of the cisterna magna** (see Chapter 10). Reported experience suggests that almost all affected fetuses demonstrate one or more of these cranial or intracranial dysmorphic features and, therefore, careful attention to these details should lead to the detection of over 95% of cases of spina bifida to complement detection of all cases of anencephaly (Table 9-2).

TABLE 9–1. *MSAFP Screening: Eastern North Carolina January 1984–December, 1988*

Total screened	44,882
First elevation	1907 (4.2%)
Repeat normal	620
Ultrasound	1287
Explained by ultrasound	−17% age correction
	−9% twins
	−4% IUFD
	−9% anomalies
Amniocentesis offered	781 (61%)

TABLE 9–2. *Cranial changes associated with spina bifida*

Cranial sign	Abnormal (No.)	Abnormal (%)
Small BPD	76/125	60.8
Frontal notching	260/268	97
Ventriculomegaly	214/286	74.8
Loss of cistern	45/66	68.2
Cerebellar Compression	183/189	96.8
Any abnormality	232/233	99.6

Modified from Watson WJ, Chescheir NC, Katz VL, Seeds JW. The role of ultrasound in evaluation of patients with elevated maternal serum alpha-fetoprotein: a review. *Obstet Gynecol* 1991;78:123.

If the patient-specific risk of a fetal ONTD based on MSAFP is reduced by only 90% (based on a conservative estimate of the sensitivity of ultrasound for the detection of ONTD), then the patient compares a significantly reduced risk of the unseen anomaly with the risk of amniocentesis. Reported experience with the use of ultrasound for the detection of ONTD supports this **enhanced complementary role** and a substantially reduced rate of invasive testing with little or no loss of diagnostic sensitivity. Some observers have suggested that amniocentesis in the evaluation of elevated MSAFP with a normal Level II ultrasound examination is now even obsolete. The role of amniocentesis should, at the very least, be a matter of patient choice after a thorough discussion of this information (Table 9-3).

Experience has shown that the rate at which patients will proceed with amniocentesis may be reduced from over 80% to under 30% when such information is provided during counseling. The skill and experience of the sonographer or so-

TABLE 9–3. *Sonographic sensitivity: spina bifida*

Author	Year	No. Screened	No. Spina Bifida	USA sensitive (%)
Campbell	1987	438	26	100
Richards	1988	609	10	80
Drugan	1988	257	12	75
Romero	1989	280	28	96
Hogge	1989	225	10	80
Katz	1990	451	15	100
Platt	1992	?	161	92
Total			262	92

Modified from Watson WJ, Chescheir NC, Katz VL, Seeds JW. The role of ultrasound in evaluation of patients with elevated maternal serum alpha-fetoprotein: a review. *Obstet Gynecol* 1991;78:123.

nologist, the inclusion of **cranial and intracranial markers** in the examination, and the **visual quality** of the images must be considered in the counseling. There is also the possibility of **fetal aneuploidy** in the absence of anomalies that must be considered. This has been estimated to be about 0.64%, not very different from expected.

ULTRASOUND AND ANEUPLOIDY SCREENING

Advanced maternal age, defined as maternal age of 35 years or more on the estimated date of delivery of a pregnancy, if used as a basis for amniocentesis, **potentially leads to the diagnosis of only 20% of all cases of Down syndrome.** Interest has grown, therefore, over the past decade in screening tests of low intrinsic risk and reasonable cost that might be applied to pregnancies in women considered historically to be at low risk for fetal aneuploidy. It is reasonable to conclude that the probability of fetal aneuploidy is increased or decreased with the presence or absence of abnormal screening test results, but it remains important for the patient to understand that the diagnosis cannot be excluded or confirmed with a screening test alone. In other words, a negative test result leaves the patient with a small residual risk, and a positive test result is not diagnostic of a fetal abnormality but only indicates increased risk for an abnormality.

SCREENING TESTS

Any screening test of low-risk patients must be considered in the context that further evaluation may require invasive testing with inherent risk to the pregnancy of some degree. Any screening test, therefore, must be judged on the basis of sensitivity, predictive value, and false-positive rate.

Sensitivity is the proportion of affected pregnancies with a positive screen. Positive predictive value is that proportion of patients with a positive screen that are actually affected. False-positive rate is that proportion of the general population that have a positive screen. The perfect test would have 100% sensitivity and virtually no false-positive results. MSAFP for ONTDs demonstrates about 85% sensitivity with about 3–4% false-positive rate.

If all patients over the age of 35 are considered the population in question, amniocentesis provides 100% sensitivity, but with a 100% false-positive rate. Maternal age as a screening test provides a sensitivity for Down syndrome of only 20%, with a predictive value of only 1/365 for the term livebirth of an affected child, or 1/270 for the diagnosis of trisomy 21 at the time of 16 week amniocentesis, with a false-positive rate of 5–8% (proportion of patients over age 35). Screening tests inevitably involve a compromise between sensitivity, predictive value, and false-positive rate. These characteristics of any screening test offered to a patient should be discussed in detail to avoid misinterpretation of either a positive or a negative result.

Maternal Serum Screening

The association between low maternal serum alpha-fetoprotein and fetal trisomy was first reported in 1984. Trisomies 13, 18, and 21 were all seen on average to show a lower MSAFP value compared with normal. Attention soon focused on trisomy 21, and the median value for Down syndrome pregnancies was found to be about 0.71 MOM of the normal population. Screening programs soon adopted a bivariant analysis based on maternal age and MSAFP value that provided diagnostic efficiency similar to that seen with advanced maternal age. MSAFP screening programs applied to women under 35, therefore, provide a sensitivity for Down syndrome of only 20–25%, and a predictive value of an abnormal screen of only 1–2%. Furthermore, it must be recalled, that trisomy 21 constitutes a diminishing proportion of the total aneuploid burden as maternal age decreases. In 20-year-old women, for instance, Down syndrome amounts to only 25–32% of the total aneuploid risk.

The observation in 1987 that maternal serum unconjugated estriol in pregnancies complicated by fetal Down syndrome (trisomy 21) is moderately depressed and, in 1989, that maternal serum quantitative human chorionic gonadotropin (HCG) is substantially increased led to the combination of all three serum markers into the **triple screen.** The use of all three maternal serum screening markers appears to offer screening sensitivity of up to 58% for fetal Down syndrome in the under-35-year population, with a predictive value of over 2% (Table 9-4). The process involves beginning with the patient's age-specific risk and applying modifiers based on each of the three serum markers to produce a unique patient-specific risk for Down syndrome. It is significant that, although depressed MSAFP is seen with all three trisomies, triple screening initially focused only on trisomy 21. More recently, significantly depressed levels of all three markers has proved useful in screening for trisomy 18.

TABLE 9–4. *MSAFP versus triple screen women under 35*

	MSAFP and age	Triple screen
Number screened	77,373	23,675
Risk cutoff	1:270	1:190
Initial positive	4.7%	6.1%
Percent offered amniocentesis	2.7%	3.2%
Percent choosing amniocentesis	2.1%	2.6%
Down syndrome cases found	18	17
Amniocenteses per case of Down syndrome	**89**	**38**
Down syndrome sensitivity	25%	58%

From Haddow JE, Palomaki GE, Knight GJ, Williams J, *et al.* Prenatal screening for Down's syndrome with use of maternal serum markers. *N Engl J Med* 1992;327:588.

TABLE 9–5. *Aneuploidy and major anomalies*

Anomaly	% Aneuploidy
Duodenal atresia	20–30
Esophageal atresia	20–30
Cardiac	40
Diaphragmatic hernia	4
G-U anomalies	20–30
Omphalocele	30–50
Cystic hygroma	70
Holoprosencephaly	40–60

ULTRASOUND SCREENING FOR FETAL ANEUPLOIDY

Major Fetal Dysmorphology

The sonographic detection of any fetal malformation should lead to consideration of fetal aneuploidy as a possible etiology and discussion of the risk/benefit balance associated with the invasive testing necessary to establish fetal karyotype. Major anomalies differ greatly in the associated risk of aneuploidy, and specific risk should be discussed (Table 9-5).

The combination of multiple anomalies substantially increases the probability of fetal aneuploidy. Paladini found congenital heart disease in 31 of 469 fetuses. Fifteen of these were aneuploid (48%); 29.4% of those with isolated heart defects proved to be aneuploid; and 71.4% of those with cardiac and noncardiac dysmorphology combined. Brown et al., reviewed 125 cases of structural cardiac anomaly detected by antenatal sonography and found 43/125 (43%) to be aneuploid overall. Aneuploidy was found in 33/52 (63%) with coexisting noncardiac anomalies, and in only 10/73 (14%) without coexisting noncardiac anomalies.

Overall, investigators have found 50% of trisomy 21 fetuses to have a major sonographic anomaly, and 90% of trisomy 13 and 18 fetuses.

SCREENING OF A LOW-RISK POPULATION

More than fifteen different forms of minor sonographic dysmorphology have been associated with fetal aneuploidy (Table 9-6).

Before any of these is used as a basis for the discussion of invasive testing, the provider should evaluate the sensitivity, predictive value, and false-positive performance of the marker.

TABLE 9–6. *Minor dysmorphic features associated with an increased risk of aneuploidy*

Limb length asymmetries
Increased nuchal skinfold thickness
Renal pyelectasis
Digital hypoplasia
Hyperechogenic bowel
Small ears
Choroid plexus cysts
Wide first toe space
Abnormal hand posturing
Micrognathia
Sloping forehead
Strawberry shaped skull
Enlarged cisterna magna
Mild ventriculomegaly
Hyperechogenic cardiac moderator band
Postaxial polydactyly
Early severe IUGR
Facial clefting

Biometric Asymmetry

Lockwood and Benacceraf described the possible utility of short femur length as a screening tool for Down syndrome in 1987. Humeral length as well has been examined as a possible screening marker for Down syndrome. Different investigators, however, using the same criteria find widely differing results (Table 9-7).

TABLE 9–7. *Limb length and Down syndrome*

Author	Marker	Sensitivity (%)	False positive (%)
Benacerraf	OFL/EFL < 0.91	68	2
Nyberg	OFL/EFL < 0.91	24.4	4.7
Perella	OFL/EFL < 0.91	28	23
Lockwood	BPD/FL > + 1.5 SD	70	7
Shah	BPD/FL > + 1.5 SD	18	6
Dicke	BPD/FL > + 1.5 SD	18	4
Benacerraf	OHu/EHu < 0.90	50	6
Rotmensch	OHu/EHu < 0.90	28	9
Nyberg	OHu/EHu < 0.90	24.4	4.5

OFL, observed femur length; EFL, expected femur length; BPD, biparietal diameter; FL, femur length; OHu, observed humerus length; EHu, expected humerus length.

Many providers do not consider mild femur length shortfall by itself to justify amniocentesis.

MINOR DYSMORPHOLOGY

Nuchal Skin Thickness

The measurement of nuchal skin thickness must be made from a carefully defined scanplane that includes the cavum septum pellucidi and the cerebellar hemispheres (Fig. 9-1). The thickness is measured outside the skull. Prior to 20 weeks gestation this should be less than 5 mm, and after 20 weeks, this should be less than 6 mm. Crane and Gray studied 3338 patients prospectively and found increased nuchal skin thickness in 12/16 (75%) of cases of Down syndrome, and only 35/3322 (1.05%) of the nonaneuploid fetuses (Fig. 9-2). A predictive value of 1/13 (7.7%) in a population with a risk of 1/710 was estimated. Expanded experience has shown the sensitivity to be closer to 40–45%, with similarly low false-positive and high predictive value. Increased nuchal skinfold thickness within a properly constructed scanplane does appear to justify discussion of further diagnostic testing.

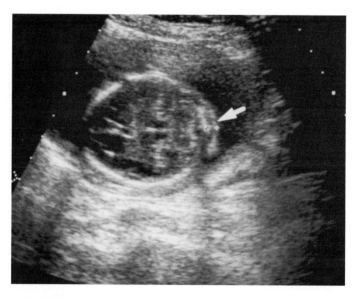

FIG. 9-1. A suboccipitobregmatic scanplane showing cavum and cerebellar hemispheres may be used to measure nuchal skin thickness. This thickness should not exceed 5 mm at less than 20 weeks.

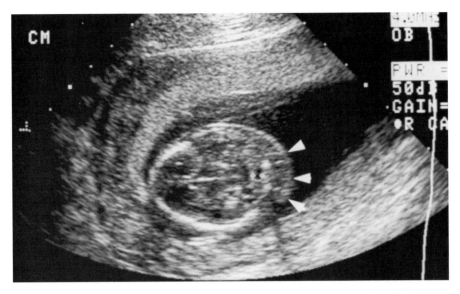

FIG. 9-2. This fetus with Down syndrome was found to have an increase in nuchal skinfold thickness *(arrowheads)*.

Renal Pyelectasis

Significant fetal renal pyelectasis has been variously defined as renal pelvis anteroposterior (AP) diameter of 4 mm or greater between 15 and 20 weeks gestation, AP diameter over 5 mm, and AP diameter over 50% of the AP diameter of the kidney in the same scanplane (Fig. 9-3A,B). Pyelectasis over 4 mm was reported by Benacerraf in 210/7400 (2.8% false-positive), and seven of these (3.3% predictive value) had Down syndrome. Among 44 fetuses with Down syndrome, 25% demonstrated mild pyelectasis (sensitivity). The need to discuss invasive testing with the patient with mild fetal renal pyelectasis remains controversial.

Digital Hypoplasia

The normal median ratio of the length of the middle phalanx of the fifth digit to that of the fourth digit in fetuses between 15 and 20 weeks gestation has been reported to be 0.85 (Fig. 9-4). A ratio of less than 0.70 has been observed to provide a sensitivity of 75%, a positive predictive value of 3.2%, and a false-positive rate of 18% for fetal Down syndrome (Fig. 9-5). Although possibly true, the practical clinical screening value of this observation is quite limited since the measurement of this parameter of the 16 week fetus is difficult and time consuming without considerable practice, and this test is not likely to gain wide practical application.

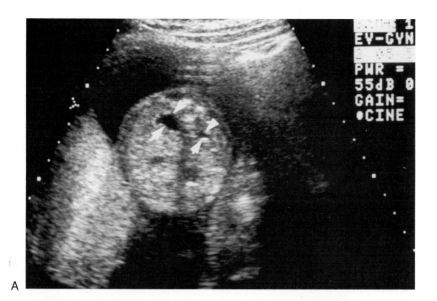

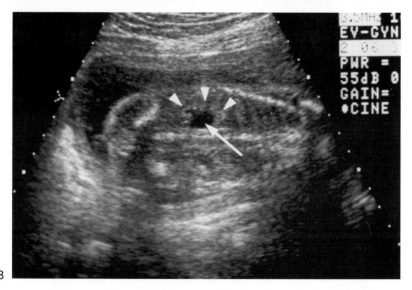

FIG. 9-3. A: Mild renal pyelectasis *(arrows),* one side greater than the other shown here on transverse view. The possibility of caliectasis cannot be adequately evaluated on this view. This fetus had Down syndrome. The only dysmorphic features found were the pyelectasis and nuchal skinfold thickening. **B:** A coronal view of the more affected kidney from (A). Note perhaps early caliectasis at the caudal end. *Long arrow,* renal pelvis.

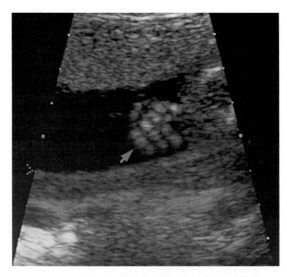

FIG. 9-4. With some practice, imaging of the fetal digits is possible. Note here the middle phalanx of the fifth digit *(arrow)* in a normal fetus and compare it with the middle phalanx of the fourth.

Hyperechogenic Bowel

Dicke and Crane identified 30/12776 (0.2%) fetuses with hyperechoic bowel, four of these were eventually diagnosed with cystic fibrosis (13.3%) and one with trisomy 18. They concluded that hyperechoic bowel was not by itself an indication for consideration of cytogenetic studies. Dubinsky et al., on the other hand,

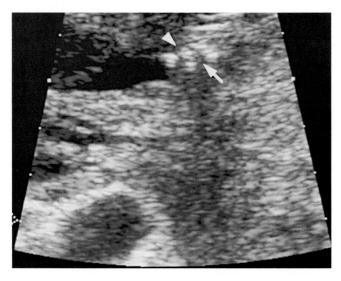

FIG. 9-5. This study demonstrates virtual absence of the middle phalanx of the fetal fifth digit *(arrow)* compared with the fourth *(arrowhead)*. Compare with the digits in Fig. 9-4.

reported abnormal outcomes in 29/64 fetuses with hyperechogenic bowel, including 14/64 (22%) with aneuploidy, mostly trisomy 21 (Fig. 9-6A,B). Hyperechogenic bowel remains, to some extent, a subjective observation (Fig. 9-7). Echogenicity equal to adjacent bone is generally proposed as the standard for discussion, but the degree of association with aneuploidy is not firmly established, and the need to discuss invasive testing does not enjoy consensus.

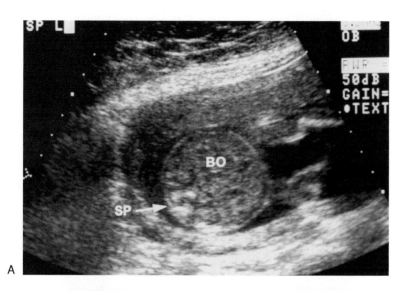

A

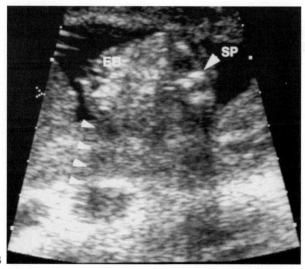

B

FIG. 9-6. A: This normal fetus shows the characteristic echotexture of bowel *(BO)*. The spine *(SP)* represents the comparative echo level. **B:** The increased echogenicity of the bowel in this fetus is apparent *(EB)*. The brightness is similar to spine *(SP),* and even demonstrates acoustic shadowing *(arrowheads).*

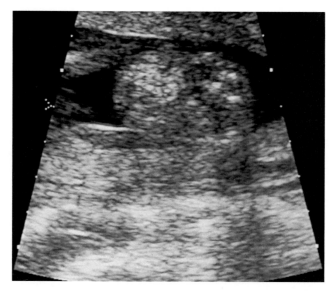

FIG. 9-7. The appreciation of echogenic bowel is subjective. Only if the bowel simulates bone in the same study, as illustrated here, is the risk of pathology sufficient to warrant discussion of any further testing.

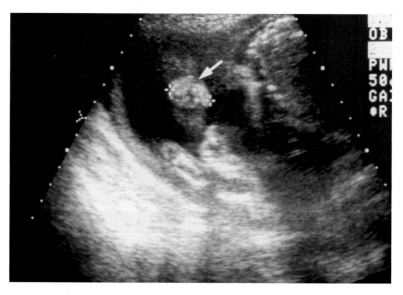

FIG. 9-8. With some practice, imaging of fetal ears is possible. This ear is clearly seen *(arrow)* and easily measured.

Small Ears

Birnholz and others have found a linear growth curve for the fetal ear described by EL = 1.1011 × EGA (wk) −9.5089 (Fig. 9-8). Short ears were found in 83% of aneuploid fetuses, all trisomy 13 and 18 (6/6), and 50% of trisomy 21 (3/6). Lettieri reported ear length data from 424 fetuses. Ear length (EL) growth was linear, and among the fourteen aneuploid fetuses, ten (71%) had EL below the tenth percentile (Fig. 9-9). The positive predictive value was, therefore, 23% and the false-positive rate 10%. Use of earlength is investigational.

Frontal Lobe Hypoplasia

Bahado-Singh et al. measured frontal lobe length (FLL), frontal lobe-cavum septum pellucidum distance (FL-CSP), and frontothalamic distance (FTD) in normal and Down syndrome infants looking specifically for frontal lobe hypoplasia. Using an observed-to-expected frontothalamic distance ratio of <0.84, their data showed a sensitivity for Down syndrome in 19 fetuses between 16 and 21 weeks gestation of 21.2%, and a predictive value of only 1.2% in a population with a prevalence of 1/270.

Choroid Plexus Cysts (CPC)

Porto found 63 cases of CPC among 3247 second trimester examinations (1.9%) between 15 and 22 weeks gestation, and of these six (9.5%) were aneu-

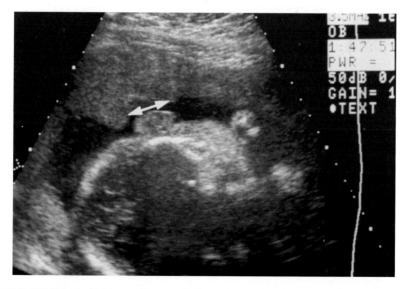

FIG. 9-9. This infant with trisomy 18 not only showed a small ear, but the shape was unusual as it extended from the side of the head.

ploid (3 trisomy 18, 2 Down, 1 Turner). The risk of aneuploidy was doubled if the diameter exceeded 5 mm (Fig. 9-10). Suessen, and others, found 109 fetuses with CPC among 11,512 patients studied. There were ten trisomy 18 fetuses, half of whom had a CPC. Ninety percent of the trisomy 18 fetuses had a major sonographic anomaly. They estimated the probability of trisomy 18 in the case of an isolated CPC to be only 1/570. Nyberg found one or more anomalies in 72% of fetuses with trisomy 18 examined before 24 weeks, and in 100% of fetuses with trisomy 18 examined after 24 weeks gestation.

Facial Clefting

Facial clefting is a common finding among fetuses with trisomies 13 and 18. However, in a study of 32 fetuses with the antenatal detection of facial clefts, although six (18.7%) were found to be aneuploid (including one trisomy 18, and five trisomy 13), in none of these was clefting isolated. Fetuses with isolated facial clefting had a good prognosis. Visualization of the fetal lips is not difficult (Fig. 9-11).

Enlarged Cisterna Magna

Enlarged cisterna magna associated with cerebellar hypoplasia was reported in 1989 in five fetuses with trisomy 18 in the third trimester (Fig. 9-12). Hill, how-

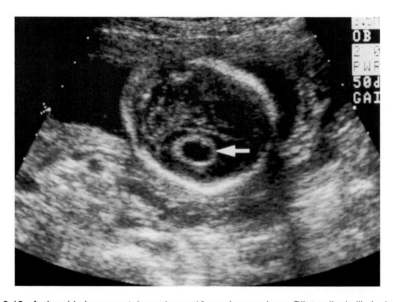

FIG. 9-10. A choroid plexus cyst *(arrow)* over 10 mm is seen here. Bilaterality is likely, but reverbation artifact from the mother or the proximal skull table often obscures the near field detail.

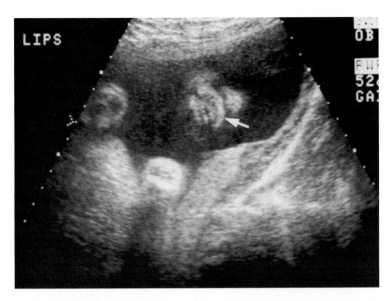

FIG. 9-11. Careful coronal scanning of the lower face will allow examination of the fetal face and lips. Clefting of the lips may be detected with such a study. Clefting of the palate without the lips is much more difficult.

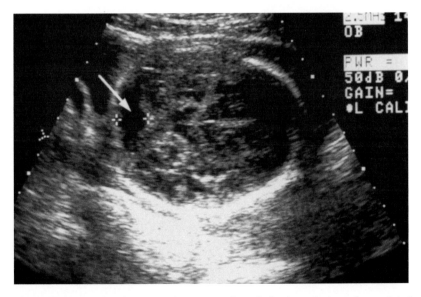

FIG. 9-12. This fetus with trisomy 18 demonstrated cerebellar hypoplasia and associated enlargement of the cisterna magna *(arrow)*. Routine imaging of the posterior fossa allows screening for such a finding, since a 10 mm cistern presents an unusual visual image.

ever, in 1991, found enlargement of the cistern in only 3/12 third-trimester fetuses with trisomy 18.

Cerebellar Hypoplasia

Eleven of 19 (58%) fetuses with trisomy 18 showed transverse cerebellar measurements more than 2 SD below the mean for gestational age. As noted above, although this observation would logically be related to enlargement of the cistern, only 3/12 infants examined in the third trimester showed enlargement of the cisterna magna.

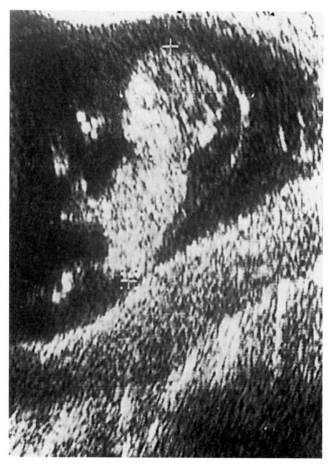

FIG. 9-13. The membrane outlining the hygroma in this 12-week fetus is easily seen and carries an ominous prognosis. Both pregnancy losses and aneuploidy are more common with such a finding.

First Trimester Cystic Hygroma

In two of eight cases of first-trimester or early second-trimester diagnosis of nuchal cystic hygroma, reported by Bronshtein et al., aneuploidy was identified (trisomy 21, and trisomy 18) (Fig. 9-13). Four of four septated hygromas were either aneuploid or ended in fetal death. Three of four nonseptated hygromas ended with normal term neonates. Another larger experience found that 7/22 fetuses found to have a cystic hygroma in the first trimester were aneuploid; four trisomy 21, two trisomy 18, and one complex abnormality. Shulman also found a high probability of aneuploidy (15/32 or 47%) among fetuses with cystic hygroma found in the first trimester but did not find that septation discriminated a good from poor outcome. Aneuploidy was found in 50% of the septate and 43% of the nonseptate. Eleven of 12 fetuses with normal chromosomal complement had a normal outcome.

OTHER OBSERVATIONS

Single Umbilical Artery

A spectrum of congenital malformations has been associated with the observation of a single umbilical artery including cardiac, neural axis, and urinary tract. Saller et al. reported retrospective data in 1990 indicating that 22% (2/9) of trisomy 18 fetuses and 33% of trisomy 13 fetuses (2/6) had a single umbilical artery, while 0/18 trisomy 21 had this observation. No prospective experience from which reliable sensitivity, predictive value, or false-positive rate might be estimated were presented.

Polyhydramnios

Damato found 7/105 patients with polyhydramnios carried aneuploid fetuses raising the question of whether polyhydramnios itself might represent an independent risk factor for fetal aneuploidy. However, all of the aneuploid fetuses demonstrated sonographic dysmorphology indicating that, in the absence of detectable anomalies, his data do not support polyhydramnios as an indication for invasive testing.

Multiple Component Scoring System

Benaceraff et al. examined major and minor dysmorphology as well as growth asymmetry demonstrated in 43 aneuploid fetuses from among 5000 14–20 week fetuses referred for examination because of advanced maternal age or abnormal MSAFP. They found that 17/32 (53%) of the Down fetuses were identified by short femur/humerus criteria, 22/32 (69%) had nuchal skin >6 mm, and 11/32

(34%) had a major anomaly. All trisomy 13/18 fetuses had a major anomaly. A scoring system giving 2 points for nuchal skin >6 mm and/or a major anomaly, and 1 point for either short long bones or renal pyelectasis, and considering **2 points as a cutoff, 81% of the Down fetuses** and 100% of the trisomy 13/18 pregnancies would be identified, with a 4.4% false-positive rate. **The predictive value for the system was estimated to be 6.87%, 3.75%, and 1.91% for risk populations of 1/250, 1/500, and 1/1000 respectively.** As experience grows with any or all of the other minor dysmorphic features associated with aneuploidy, they may be added to this scoring system and given appropriate status. Some alone justify consideration of invasive testing, while others justify further testing only in combination.

SUMMARY

Clearly ultrasound plays a critical complementary role to maternal serum screening for many congenital anomalies or conditions. With elevated MSAFP, ultrasound may provide a benign explanation or identify one of several malformations that might cause the elevation. If no explanation is found, the demonstrated sensitivity of ultrasound may be helpful to the patient in considering further testing.

In the case of low MSAFP or an abnormal multiple marker screen, ultrasound may provide additional information supporting an increased risk of aneuploidy. Furthermore, if, in the course of an obstetric ultrasound examination, a major anomaly, a first trimester hygroma, nuchal skin thickness in excess of 5 mm, or a combination of short limbs and mild pyelectasis, or severe early IUGR is noted, consideration of fetal karyotyping may be appropriate.

Ultrasound is inherently subjective in its performance. The care and experience necessary to provide the diagnostic sensitivities discussed here are not always available. Even under ideal circumstances, ultrasound cannot make or exclude the diagnosis of fetal aneuploidy. About 6 of every 1000 liveborn infants has a chromosomal abnormality (aneuploidy). The rate rises slowly with maternal age. Of the 120 cytogenetic disorders expected in 20,000 live births, 25 cases of trisomy 21 (Down syndrome), 2–3 cases of trisomy 18, and 1 infant with trisomy 13 would be found. Fewer than 25% of the cases of trisomy 21 are born to women over age 35. Open neural tube defects (ONTDs) complicate 1–2 per thousand livebirths in the United States. The rate varies somewhat by region and race and is substantially increased with insulin-dependent diabetes. MSAFP screening aimed at the detection of ONTDs has been an accepted element of antenatal care since 1985. Triple serum screening for the detection of fetal aneuploidy is growing in acceptance. Ultrasound complements both types of screening. Elevated MSAFP can lead to the identification of **85%** of the 1–2/1000 pregnancies complicated by a fetal **open neural tube defect (ONTD), ventral wall defect, and urinary tract anomaly associated with severe oligohydramnios.** Low MSAFP can lead to the detection of 20% of those pregnancies complicated by fetal trisomy 21; **triple screening may allow the detection of up to 58% of these.** **Ultrasound** confirms **gestational age, fetal number,** and **viability,** and has been shown capable of detection of over **95% of ONTDs,** as well as the most ventral wall and urinary tract anomalies. **Ultrasound** can detect growth asymmetries as well as many major and **minor fetal dysmorphologies** associated with fetal aneuploidy. The majority of aneuploid fetuses are **morphologically different** and **the greater the number of dysmorphic features the higher the probability of aneuploidy.** Ultrasound **cannot make or exclude** the diagnosis of fetal aneuploidy, but a careful search for both major and minor markers clearly may increase or decrease risk.

FURTHER READING

Adams MJ, Windham GC, Greenberg JF, *et al.* Clinical interpretation of maternal serum alpha-fetoprotein concentrations. *Am J Obstet Gynecol* 1984;148:241.

Bahado-Singh RO, Wyse L, Dorr MA, *et al.* Fetuses with Down syndrome have disproportionately shortened frontal lobe dimensionos on ultrasonographic examination. *Am J Obstet Gynecol* 1992;167:1009.

Benacerraf BR, Barss VA, Laboda LA. A sonographic sign for the detection in the second trimester of the fetus with Down's syndrome. *Am J Obstet Gynecol* 1985;151:1078.

Benacerraf BR, Gelman R, Frigoletto FD. Sonographic identification of second-trimester fetuses with Down's syndrome. *N Engl J Med* 1987;317:1371.

Benacerraf BR, Harlow BL, Frigoletto FD. Hypoplasia of the middle phalanx of the fifth digit. *J Ultrasound Med* 1990;9:389.

Benacerraf BR, Laboda LA. Cyst of the fetal choroid plexus: a normal varient? *Am J Obstet Gynecol* 1989;160:319.

Benacerraf BR, Mandell J, Estroff JA, Harlow BL, Frigoletto FD. Fetal pyelectasis: a possible association with Down syndrome. *Obstet Gynecol* 1990;76:58.

Benacerraf BR, Neuberg D, Bromley B, Frigoletto FD. Sonographic scoring index for prenatal detection of chromosomal abnormalities. *J Ultrasound Med* 1992;11:449.

Benacerraf BR, Neuberg D, Frigoletto FD. Humeral shortening in second-trimester fetuses with Down syndrome. *Obstet Gynecol* 1991;77:223.

Birnholz JC, Farrell EE. Fetal ear length. *Pediatrics* 1988;81:555.

Bronshtein M, Rottem S, Yoffe N, Blumenfeld Z. First trimester and early second trimester diagnosis of nuchal cystic hygroma by transvaginal sonography: diverse prognosis of the septated from the nonseptated lesion. *Am J Obstet Gynecol* 1989;161:78–82.

Crane JP, Gray DL. Sonographically measured nuchal skinfold thickness as a screening tool for Down syndrome: results of a prospective clinical trial. *Obstet Gynecol* 1991;77:533.

Dicke JM, Gray DL, Songster GS, *et al.* Fetal biometry as a screening tool for the detection of chromosomally abnormal pregnancies. *Obstet Gynecol* 1989;74:726.

Dicke JM, Crane JP. Sonographically detected hyperechoic fetal bowel: significance and implications for pregnancy management. *Obstet Gynecol* 1992;80:778.

Drugan A, Zador IE, Syner FN, *et al.* A normal ultrasound does not obviate the need for amniocentesis in patients with elevated serum alpha-fetoprotein. *Obstet Gynecol* 1988;72:627.

Dubinsky TJ, Nyberg DA, Mahony BS, *et al.* Hyperechogenic fetal bowel: clinical significance. *J Ultrasound Med* 1993;12:S55.

Haddow JE, Palomaki GE, Knight GJ, Williams J, *et al.* Prenatal screening for Down's syndrome with use of maternal serum markers. *N Engl J Med* 1992;327:588.

Hill LM, Marchese S, Peterson C, Fries J. The effect of trisomy 18 on transverse cerebellar diameter. *Am J Obstet Gynecol* 1991;165:72.

Hook EB. Rates of chromosome abnormalities at different maternal ages. *Obstet Gynecol* 1981;58:282.

Lettieri L, Rodis JF, Vintzileos AM, *et al.* Ear length in second-trimester aneuploid fetuses. *Obstet Gynecol* 1993;81:57.

Macri JN, Haddow JE, Weiss RR. Screening for neural tube defects in the United States: A summary of the Scarborough Conference. *Am J Obstet Gynecol* 1979;133:119.

Perrella R, Duerinckx AJ, Grant EG, *et al.* Second-trimester sonographic diagnosis of Down syndrome: role of femur-length shortening and nuchal-fold thickening. *AJR* 1988;151:981.

Paladini D, Calabro R, Palmieri S, D'Andrea T. Prenatal diagnosis of congenital heart disease and fetal karyotyping. *Obstet Gynecol* 1993;81:679.

Platt LD, Feuchtbaum L, Filly R, *et al.* The California Maternal Serum AlphaFetoprotein Screening Program: the role of ultrasonography in the detection of spina bifida. *Am J Obstet Gynecol* 1992;166:1328.

Porto M, Murata Y, Warneke LA, Keegan KA. Fetal choroid plexus cysts: an independent risk factor for chromsomal anomalies. *J Clin Ultrasound* 1993;21:103.

Shah YG, Eckl CJ, Stinson SK, *et al.* Biparietal diameter/femur length ratio, cephalic index and femur length measurements: not reliable screening techniques for Down syndrome. *Obstet Gynecol* 1990;75:186.

Shulman LP, Emerson DS, Felker RE, *et al.* High frequency of cytogenetic abnormalities in fetuses with cystic hygroma diagnosed in the first trimester. *Obstet Gynecol* 1992;80:80.

van Zalen-Sprock RM, van Vugt JMG, van Geijn HP. First trimester diagnosis of cystic hygroma—course and outcome. *Am J Obstet Gynecol* 1992;167:94.

Watson WJ, Chescheir NC, Katz VL, Seeds JW. The role of ultrasound in evaluation of patients with elevated maternal serum alpha-fetoprotein: a review. *Obstet Gynecol* 1991;78:123.

10

Sonographic Diagnosis of Malformations of the Central Nervous System

The central nervous system (CNS) is the second most likely site of an isolated malformation after the heart and also a common site of malformation associated with aneuploidy or syndromic conditions. Although congenital malformations of any major fetal organ system may be associated with significant developmental disabilities, disproportionate attention has been focused on malformations of the central nervous system perhaps because both mental and motor function may be impaired.

Malformations that affect the central nervous system are varied in type and appearance. Both neural tube and non-neural tube defects may be identified with antenatal ultrasound, and a variety of axial defects near the neural tube may also be found. The screening examination of the fetal neural system should be methodical and complete and no observation, no matter how obvious, may be taken for granted.

NORMAL CENTRAL NERVOUS SYSTEM

The shape and size of the cranium, the presence of midline membranes, the size of lateral ventricles, and the integrity of the posterior fossa are all important elements of the screening examination. None of these routine observations can be taken for granted.

The standard **occipitofrontal** scanplane from which a biparietal diameter **(BPD)** is typically measured is a good starting point. An easy starting point is to align the scanplane with the fetal spine, slide up to the cranium, then rotate the transducer 90 degrees. Typically, this maneuver will produce a nearly transaxial occipitofrontal image. The cranial outline should be oval and uniform in shape; a midline should be apparent. The **cavum septum pellucidum** is seen in the midline just ahead of the **thalami,** and the lateral ventricles are seen both at the

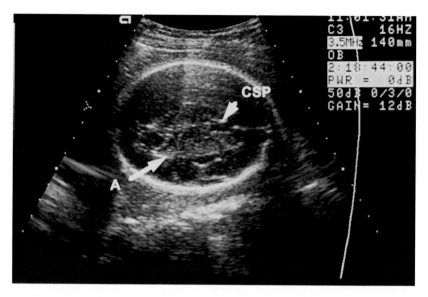

FIG. 10-1. The occipitofrontal scanplane perpendicular to the midline allows an assessment of the oval shape, the midline, the cavum septum pellucidum *(CSP),* and the atrium *(A)* of the lateral ventricle. The cavum is just ahead of and the atrium just lateral and behind the thalami. All of these seemingly casual observations are important in screening for unexpected malformation.

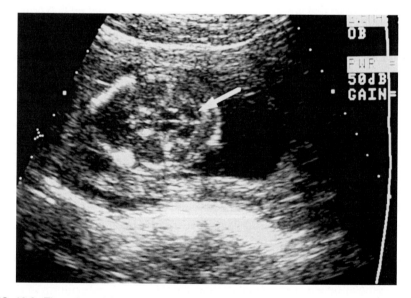

FIG. 10-2. The atrium of the lateral ventricle should be measured across the tail of the choroid as illustrated here. The correct dimension does not include wall thickness and is measured perpendicular to the axis of the ventricle, not perpendicular to the midline. The atrium should not exceed 10 mm.

frontal horns and the **atria** (Fig. 10-1). The choroid plexus normally fills the atrium of the lateral ventricle, but, in about 5% of patients, a fluid space is seen between the choroid and the medial ventricular wall. The lateral ventricular width across the choroid at the **atrium** should be less than 10 mm, measuring only the lumen at a right angle to the axis of the ventricle (Fig. 10-2).

The **posterior fossa** should be found within a suboccipitobregmatic plane, produced from the occipitofrontal scanplane by rotating the occipital heel of the transducer slightly caudally. The standard posterior fossa view will contain both **cerebellar hemispheres** and the cavum (Fig. 10-3). The cerebellar hemispheres are seen to be symmetric and circular. Fluid should be clearly seen within the **cisterna magna,** and **nuchal skin thickness** dorsal to the midline occipital skull may be measured.

The fetal spine may be imaged in both longitudinal and transverse views and there are five distinct longitudinal views (Fig. 10-4A,B). The oblique longitudinal view was popular for some time probably because it typically provided a complete image of the ventrally flexed fetal spine (Fig. 10-5). Unfortunately, the oblique view is less sensitive to small dysraphic defects and is, therefore, not recommended. The coronal view, although imposing the need to develop several sequential images in order to completely capture the same ventrally flexed fetal spine, provides a more sensitive examination.

Transverse views of the fetal spine prior to 20 weeks show three echocenters

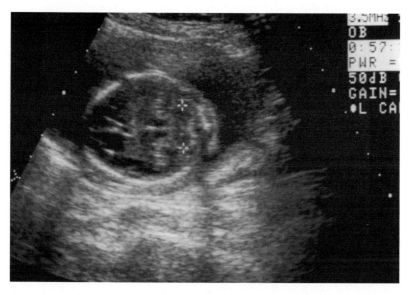

FIG. 10-3. A modest caudal rotation of the occipital heel of the transducer from the view in FIG. 10-2 should bring the posterior fossa into view. The cerebellar hemispheres should present a circular and symmetric appearance *(between cursors),* and there should appear a fluid (anechoic) layer in the cisterna magna dorsal to the hemispheres. It is from this view, with cavum and cerebellar hemispheres in the same plane, that skin thickness dorsal to the cranial vault may be measured as a screening tool for Down syndrome.

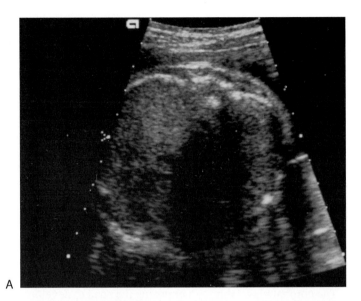

A

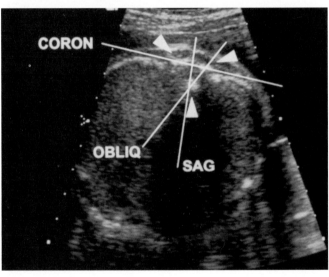

B

FIG. 10-4. A: Just to the right of center at the top of this transverse abdominal view, the three echocenters *(bright spots)* that constitute the sonographic appearance of the normal fetal transverse spine may be seen. The dense acoustic shadow beneath the spine is characteristic. **B:** Possible longitudinal scanplanes drawn through the spinal echocenters may be sagittal, one of two obliques, and either a deep or very superficial coronal. The coronal illustrated here is the most sensitive of the longitudinal scanplanes.

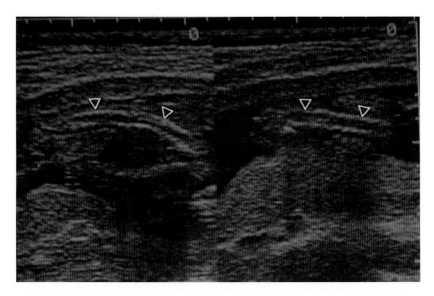

FIG. 10-5. The oblique longitudinal, on the left, was once more popular since it is easier to capture more of the gently ventrally flexed fetal spine *(arrows)* in one scanplane. However, the coronal, on the right, is the more sensitive of the two examinations. (*Source:* Reprinted from Seeds JW, Azizkhan RG. *Congenital Malformations: Antenatal Diagnosis, Perinatal Management, and Counseling.* Rockville, MD: Aspen Publishers Inc., ©1990; p. 80.)

that correlate roughly with the vertebral body ventrally and the neural arches dorsally. Sweeping the transducer throughout the length of the spine from cranium to sacrum in the transverse orientation will allow the examiner to evaluate the geometric relationship of these echocenters. The three echocenters should maintain a constant relationship to one another throughout the length. Coronal longitudinal and transverse spinal views should be developed to show normal orderly spinal anatomy throughout its length.

The basic, or office ultrasound examination should include a screening examination of the fetal central nervous system that demonstrates the anatomy listed in Table 10-1. Features of shape, symmetry, midline, ventricles, posterior fossa, and spinal anatomy should be addressed.

TABLE 10–1. *Standard CNS views*

Occipitofrontal transaxial
Shape and size
Atrial width
Cavum
Posterior fossa (suboccipitobregmatic)
Cerebellar shape
Cistern
Nuchal skin
Coronal longitudinal spine
Transverse spine

MALFORMATIONS OF THE CENTRAL NERVOUS SYSTEM

Initiation of the process that ultimately results in the diagnosis of a malformation of the central nervous system is typically based on the detection of a deviation from the expected normal appearance of one or more of the elements of the examination outlined above. Often, malformations are visually prominent, and it is obvious to the examiner that normal anatomy is absent. Sometimes, though, minor sorts of observations lead to the diagnosis of a more subtle abnormality. Detectable CNS anomalies are found in Table 10-2.

Failure to diagnose a major malformation of the central nervous system is often the result of an incomplete examination, not the subtle nature of the defect. Furthermore, the identification of one defect should immediately raise the possibility of another, such as spina bifida related to hydrocephalus. Once a malformation is adequately characterized, a careful search for others should begin.

Deviations from the normal, expected anatomy and possible diagnostic associations are listed in Table 10-3.

Open Neural Tube Defects (ONTDs)

The neural ridges begin to develop on the dorsum of the embryonic disc about 18 days after conception, grow together, and fuse first in the thoracic region forming a neural tube, with fusion spreading up and down simultaneously to closure of the posterior neuropore at about 26 days post conception. Failure of closure at either end results in a neural tube defect. Caudal ONTDs (spina bifida) occur with about equal frequency as cranial open neural tube defects (anencephaly) (Table 10-4).

Neural tube defects were expected in 1–2 per thousand live births in the United States prior to widespread population screening programs. About half of these are cranial and about half spinal. About 95% of ONTDs occur **with no family history.** The birth of such a child, however, is associated with a 2–4% probability of recurrence within a family. Recurrence may be in the form of any of several types of neural tube defects. Several large studies have shown that folate sup-

---

TABLE 10–2. *Potentially detectable anomalies*

Hydrocephalus
Holoprosencephaly
Dandy-Walker malformation
Porencephaly
Anencephaly
Spina bifida
Encephalocele
Cystic hygroma
Facial clefting
Teratomas

TABLE 10–3. *Diagnosis resulting from sonographic screening*

Sonographic finding	Possible diagnosis
Frontal notching	Spina bifida
Mild ventriculomegaly	Spina bifida
	Down syndrome
	Hydrocephalus
Absent cavum	Agenesis of corpus callosum
Cerebellar compression	Spina bifida
Absent cisterna magna	Spina bifida
Nuchal skin > 5 mm thick	Down syndrome
Spinal dysraphism	Spina bifida
Absent midline	Holoprosencephaly
	Hydranencephaly
Severe ventriculomegaly	Extreme hydrocephalus
	Hydranencephaly
Dilatation of 4th ventricle	Dandy-Walker malformation
Irregular anechoic areas	Porencephalic cysts
Frontal cranial defect	Frontal encephalocele
Occipital cranial defect	Occipital encephalocele
Extreme dorsiflexion of occiput	Iniencephaly
Solid/cystic masses of sacrum	Sacrococcygeal teratoma

plementation prior to conception lowers incidence by at least 50% and recurrence by up to 75%, even though folate deficiency by any traditional standard does not exist in these patients. These incidence and recurrence patterns are characteristic of congenital malformations classified as multifactorial or polygenic in origin.

Neural tube defects have been the focus of intense research and diagnostic interest for over two decades. Recognition of the association between elevated amniotic fluid and maternal serum alphafetoprotein levels and open neural tube defects led to the development of maternal serum alphafetoprotein (MSAFP) screening programs for the detection of ONTDs in early pregnancy (see Chapter 9). MSAFP is elevated in about 85% of pregnancies complicated by a fetal ONTD, and an ultrasound examination is normally the next evaluation of a pregnancy with an elevated MSAFP to confirm gestational age, fetal number, and fetal viability. As well, diagnosis of malformations may be accomplished by personnel who are trained and experienced in their detection.

TABLE 10–4. *Types of ONTD*

Anencephaly
Occipital cephalocele
Frontal cephalocele
Spina bifida
Iniencephaly

Anencephaly

Anencephaly constitutes about half of all ONTDs, and should be detected with ultrasound 100% of the time after 14-weeks gestation. Examples of earlier diagnosis are common, but the diagnostic sensitivity of earlier detection is not proved. Absence of the cranium is the basis of the diagnosis (Fig. 10-6). Variable amounts of neural soft tissue may be seen arising from the base of the skull, but most often, the spine ends abruptly above the chest, and only the base of the skull and the face are detectable.

Anencephaly is a lethal defect, but the time of death and the length of life cannot be precisely determined. Anencephalics may die *in utero,* during labor, in the neonatal period, and, rarely, later in the infantile period. Occasionally, anencephalics go home. The possibility of some variable length of life should be mentioned upon diagnosis.

The sonographic diagnosis is made upon failure to identify a fetal cranium despite a careful search. False-negative diagnosis should be rare or nonexistent. False-positive diagnosis may occasionally occur in the case of deep pelvic engagement of the vertex and an obese patient causing poor quality of images. In such a case, endovaginal scanning is mandatory to confirm the diagnosis. Typically, the rest of the fetal anatomic screen is negative, and the fetus is most often very active. Late in pregnancy, polyhydramnios is a common finding, gen-

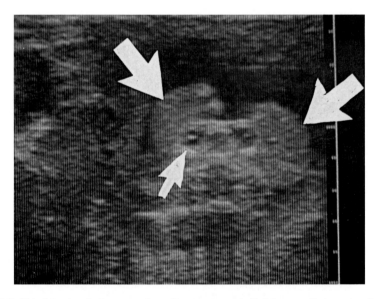

FIG. 10-6. This fetus is missing a cranium. Some anencephalic fetuses will show development of some soft tissue from the base of the skull as seen here *(large arrows). (Source:* Reprinted from Seeds JW, Azizkhan RG. *Congenital Malformations: Antenatal Diagnosis, Perinatal Management, and Counseling.* Rockville, MD: Aspen Publishers Inc, ©1990; p. 81.)

erally held to result from defective secretion of antidiuretic hormone by the impaired hypophysis.

Spina Bifida

About half of ONTDs occur in the form of spina bifida. Craniospinal rachischisis represents the most severe, complete failure of closure along the entire length of the neural tube (Fig. 10-7), but, fortunately, this form of neural tube defect is rare. Lumbar, lumbosacral, and sacral spina bifida represents the majority of caudal neural tube defects. The sonographic diagnosis of spina bifida involves both a direct longitudinal and transverse examination of the fetal spine, and a careful examination of cranial and intracranial anatomy.

The direct sonographic examination of the fetal spine in the early second trimester is generally expected to lead to diagnosis of about 75–80% of cases of OSB (open spina bifida) if performed by trained and experienced personnel. Optimal diagnostic sensitivity is found only if both serial transverse and longitudinal scanning is performed. Careful attention to the geometric relationship of the three primary echocenters to one another, as well as to the integrity of the soft tissue dorsal to them on transverse scanning is required. At least five different longitudinal views are possible. Either one of two oblique longitudinal views are typically popular because of the relative ease with which the entire ventrally

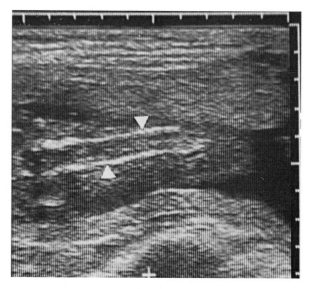

FIG. 10-7. This coronal view of the dorsal echocenters of this fetal spine show parallel but wide separation. This neural tube *(arrowheads)* failed to close throughout its length, indicating craniospinal rachyschisis.

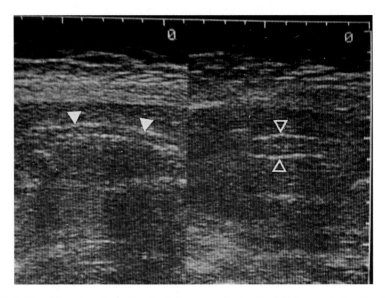

FIG. 10-8. The oblique longitudinal on the left appeared normal, while the coronal on the right of the same fetus showed a subtle divergence of echocenters that indicated spina bifida. (*Source:* Seeds JW, Azizkhan RG. *Congenital Malformations: Antenatal Diagnosis, Perinatal Management, and Counseling.* Rockville, MD: Aspen Publishers Inc, ©1990; p. 87.)

flexed fetal spine may be captured. Unfortunately, the oblique view is the least sensitive of all to small dysraphic lesions (Fig. 10-8).

Coronal views are a bit more difficult, because several sequential coronal views are required to survey the entire fetal spine due to the normal, gentle, ventral flexure. However, the coronal views are required to produce optimal diagnostic sensitivity for small defects. A superficial coronal view may be very revealing when available, but it is the distinct minority of cases in which such a view is available (Fig. 10-9).

On transverse scan in the area of the spinal defect, the dorsal paramedian echocenters are seen to be separated, and the soft tissue dorsal to the affected segments disrupted (Fig. 10-10). Often a thin-walled sac containing either fluid alone or fluid with soft tissue or membranes is seen dorsal to the defect. The spine may or may not appear angulated in the area of the defect. Longitudinal scanning shows a fusiform divergence of the echocenters in the area of the defect, most pronounced in the coronal views.

FIG. 10-10. Later gestation, diagnosis may be less difficult. Here, the transverse view on the left indicates a separation of the dorsal enters *(open arrow)*. On the right the *triangles* point to the divergent centers supporting the diagnosis. (*Source:* Reprinted from Seeds JW, Azizkhan RG. *Congenital Malformations: Antenatal Diagnosis, Perinatal Management, and Counseling.* Rockville, MD: Aspen Publishers Inc, ©1990; p. 90.)

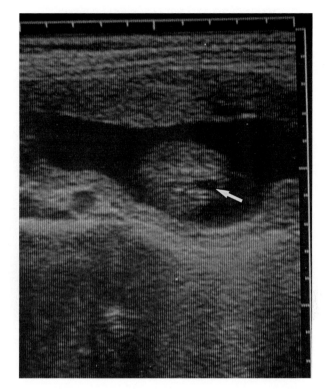

FIG. 10-9. A superficial coronal view of the skin defect associated with the findings in Fig. 10-8 confirming a small spina bifida. (*Source:* Reprinted from Seeds JW, Azizkhan RG. *Congenital Malformations: Antenatal Diagnosis, Perinatal Management, and Counseling.* Rockville, MD: Aspen Publishers Inc, ©1990; p. 89.)

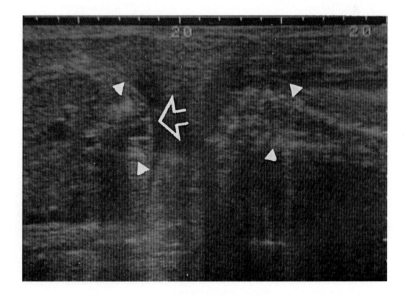

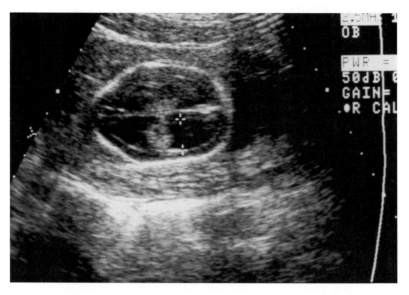

FIG. 10-11. This cranial shape is not uniformly oval, but pointed at the frontal end (lemon sign). Furthermore, mild ventriculomegaly is illustrated. If the BPD were apparent, it would be 1–2 weeks behind dates and other fetal measurements.

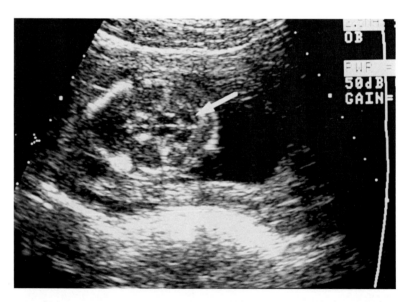

FIG. 10-12. The Chiari II malformation associated with spina bifida results from a tethering of the cord and a compression and tension pulling the cerebellar hemispheres to and into the foramen magnum. The distortion illustrated here (banana sign, *arrow*) of the cerebellar hemispheres is typical. Note also the obliteration of the cisterna magna.

Cranial changes associated with spina bifida were first described by Campbell in 1987 and confirmed since by many investigators. The five cranial changes associated with spina bifida include frontoparietal notching (lemon sign) (Fig. 10-11), mild ventriculomegaly (12–15 mm at the atrium), small biparietal diameter for dates (1–2 weeks), cerebellar compression deformities (banana sign) (Fig. 10-12), and absent cisterna magna (Fig. 10-13A,B). The posterior fossa findings are

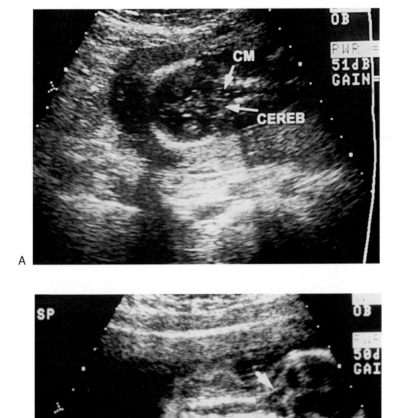

FIG. 10-13. A: A coronal view of a normal posterior fossa shows the normal circular cerebellar hemispheres *(CEREB)* over the foramen magnum and the cervical spine. Fluid fills the cisterna magna *(CM).* **B:** The cerebellar hemispheres in the case of spina bifida are pulled into the upper cervical spine as seen here *(arrow).* Compare with (A).

TABLE 10–5. *Cranial changes associated with spina bifida*

Cranial sign	Abnormal (no./total no.)	Abnormal (%)
Small BPD	76/125	60.8
Frontal notching	260/268	97
Ventriculomegaly	214/286	74.8
Loss of cistern	45/66	68.2
Cerebellar compression	183/189	96.8
Any abnormality	**232/233**	**99.6**

the antenatal sonographic equivalent of the Chiari II deformity that virtually all babies with spina bifida demonstrate (Table 10-5).

Review of published experience suggests that well over 95% of fetuses with OSB will demonstrate one or more of the above cranial changes. A similar review of overall diagnostic experience with sonography and spina bifida will show that over 90% of cases are detectable (Table 10-6). If 100% of anencephalic cases are detectable and over 90% of spina bifida are detectable then overall sonographic diagnostic sensitivity for open neural tube defects should be over 95%.

Cephaloceles

Cephaloceles may be frontal or occipital, and are often skin covered. The occipital encephalocele typically contains some soft tissue (Fig. 10-14) but may be entirely fluid filled (Fig. 10-15). Cephaloceles may be associated with intracranial ventriculomegaly or not, micro- or macrocephaly, or normal cranial growth and proportions. The prognosis for the infant is profoundly better in the case of a fluid-filled encephalocele with normal ventricles and normal cranial proportions than it is with abnormalities of ventricle or proportions.

TABLE 10–6. *Sonographic sensitivity: Spina bifida*

Author	Year	No. screened	No. Spina bifida	USA sensitive (%)
Campbell	1987	438	26	100
Richards	1988	609	10	80
Drugan	1988	257	12	75
Romero	1989	280	28	96
Hogge	1989	225	10	80
Katz	1990	451	15	100
Platt	1992	?	161	92
Total			**262**	**92**

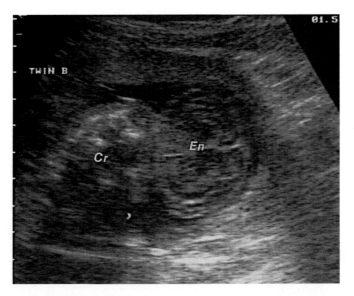

FIG. 10-14. A large occipital encephalocele filled with soft tissue (En) and associated with microcephaly (Cr). The prognosis in such a case is very poor. (*Source:* Reprinted from Seeds JW, Azizkhan RG. *Congenital Malformations: Antenatal Diagnosis, Perinatal Management, and Counseling.* Rockville, MD: Aspen Publishers Inc, ©1990; p. 84.)

Iniencephaly

Debate continues about the origins and true developmental nature of iniencephaly. The condition involves cervical spinal dysraphic changes, severe dorsiflexion of the head, and fusion of the occiput to the cervical spinal segments. There is not consensus that iniencephaly represents a true neural tube defect. Most often associated with fetal or neonatal death, occasional infants may be salvaged with surgical release of the fusion and repair of the defect.

Lipomyelomeningocele

A teratoma of the cauda equina, attaching the terminal spinal cord to a subcutaneous fatty tumor through perhaps a secondary dysraphic defect of the lower spine, this defect too sparks debate about whether it is truly a neural tube defect or primarily an unlucky teratoma. The only external finding is the subcutaneous fatty tumor over the lower spinal midline. The tumor is typically fluctuant and harmless looking, and most often the infant is neurologically intact at birth. However, failure to recognize the nature of the tumor and failure to properly remove it can lead to neurologic damage as the infant grows and the tethering of the cord results in an ascending neuropathy.

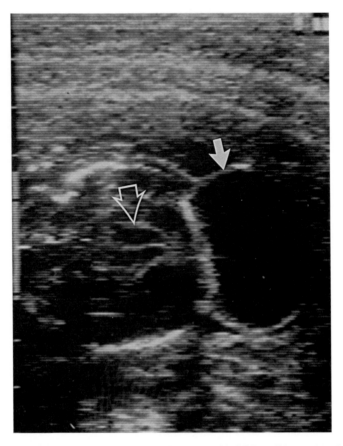

FIG. 10-15. A large occipital encephalocele filled only with CSF *(solid arrow)* and associated with normal cranial dimensions may have a good prognosis. *Open arrow,* brainstem. (*Source:* Reprinted from Seeds JW, Azizkhan RG. *Congenital Malformations: Antenatal Diagnosis, Perinatal Management, and Counseling.* Rockville, MD: Aspen Publishers Inc, ©1990; p. 82.)

The sonographic appearance is that of an echogenic subcutaneous tumor over the lower spine, with separation of the dorsal spinal segments in the area. Anechoic areas within the tumor representing a meningocele may or may not be seen.

Holoprosencephaly

Failure of the prosencephalon to divide in the 8th week and form bilateral cerebral hemispheres results in a single cerebrum with a single cerebral ventricle (Fig. 10-16). A spectrum of appearance is seen in the fetus and neonate from near normal appearance to severe malformation with variable survival and func-

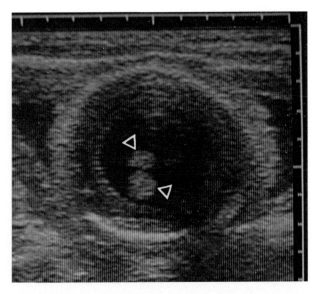

FIG. 10-16. The *open triangles* indicate the paired choroid plexes within a single cerebral ventricle in a fetus with holoprosencephaly. Typically microcephalic, survival may be roughly predicted by a careful examination of facial anatomy. (*Source:* Reprinted from Seeds JW, Azizkhan RG. *Congenital Malformations: Antenatal Diagnosis, Perinatal Management, and Counseling.* Rockville, MD: Aspen Publishers Inc, ©1990; p. 113.)

tional prognosis. Since many facial features are, in fact, induced in development by the normal development of bilateral cranial nerves, the abnormal brain development is often associated with abnormal facial features. Prognosis is roughly related to facial anatomy. Survival is more likely, though typically with disabilities, in the case of a near normal looking face. Single orbits, narrow-spaced eyes, or even a proboscis in place of a nose are often seen. There is a very increased risk of aneuploidy with holoprosencephaly.

Hydranencephaly

Absence of cerebral tissue with an intact cranium is called hydranencephaly. The brainstem and posterior fossa may be variably preserved. The cranium is completely filled with anechoic cerebral spinal fluid (CSF) (Fig. 10-17), and is linked to an early vascular accident of the internal carotid arteries with subsequent resorption of cerebral tissues. Most often, membranes are preserved, including a midline, and craniomegaly is common but not universal. Survival for variable periods is likely but neurobehavioral development is not possible. Confirmation of diagnosis antenatally may require tomography or magnetic resonance imaging.

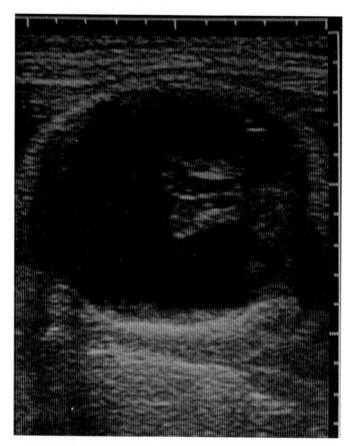

FIG. 10-17. Hydranencephaly is a condition associated with bilateral internal carotid artery occlusion. No cortical mantle is found within the cranium, although paired thalami are seen. (*Source:* Reprinted from Seeds JW, Azizkhan RG. *Congenital Malformations: Antenatal Diagnosis, Perinatal Management, and Counseling.* Rockville, MD: Aspen Publishers Inc, ©1990; p. 112.)

Dandy-Walker Malformation

Obstruction of foramina of Luschka or Magendie results in dilatation of the 4th ventricle and secondary supratentorial hydrocephalus. The 4th ventricle cyst may be small (Fig. 10-18), or profound (Fig. 10-19). Generally Dandy-Walker carries a poorer neurobehavioral prognosis than isolated hydrocephalus due to an aqueductal obstruction.

Arachnoid Cyst

Delamination and arachnoid cyst formation may occur in many locations and produce asymmetric and confusing anatomic deformation (Fig. 10-20).

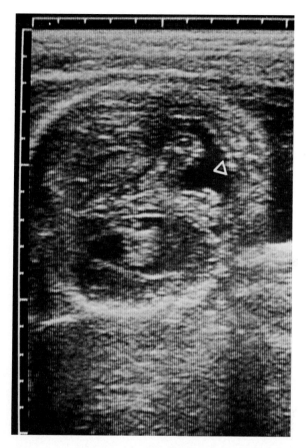

FIG. 10-18. The *open triangle* indicates an anechoic separation of the cerebellar hemispheres that is a Dandy-Walker malformation. The apparent communication of the fourth ventricle with the cistern is a deception. The obstruction of the foramena of Luschka and Magendie results in elevation of the roof of the fourth ventricle and obliteration of the cistern.

Prognosis varies from very good to poor and cannot be precisely assessed antenatally.

Sacrococcygeal Teratoma (SCT)

Teratomas may arise anywhere, including the sacrum. SCTs may be internal (Fig. 10-21) or external, cystic or solid (Fig. 10-22) or both. Typically, a sacrococcygeal teratoma presents a poorly organized, mixed pattern of cystic and soft-tissue texture. SCTs may be resected with no residual disability or with disability depending on size and location, and, if completely internal and undiagnosed in early infancy, do show a malignant potential.

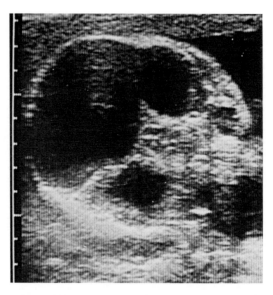

FIG. 10-19. A severe form of Dandy-Walker malformation with complete obliteration of recognizable soft tissue structures in the posterior fossa.

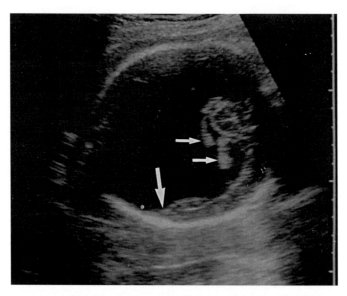

FIG. 10-20. Bizarre and unusual anatomy characterizes arachnoid cysts. Here, the cyst has divided the cortical hemispheres. The *large arrow* indicates the extent of cortex half way up the inside of the cranium. The cyst fills the cranium. The choroids dangle within the dilated ventricle. (*Source:* Reprinted from Seeds JW, Azizkhan RG. *Congenital Malformations: Antenatal Diagnosis, Perinatal Management, and Counseling.* Rockville, MD: Aspen Publishers Inc, ©1990; p. 120.)

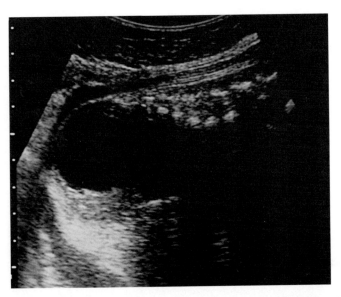

FIG. 10-21. Follow the spinal elements to the left and find the anechoic mass filling the pelvis of this fetus. This is an internal cystic sacrococcygeal teratoma. At birth, only a modest bulging of the perineum was seen.

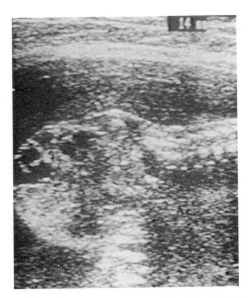

FIG. 10-22. This disorganized cystic and solid mass arising from the distal spine is a solid, external sacrococcygeal teratoma. These masses must be handled gently to avoid even minimal trauma because large vascular supply is very fragile, and life-threatening hemorrhage is possible.

Nuchal Teratoma

Cervical spinal teratomas also present a mixed appearance, most often mixed cystic/solid (Fig. 10-23). These may result in immediate neonatal ventilatory emergencies and be resectable only with difficulty but are most often survivable. Teratomas may even arise under the tongue (Fig. 10-24). A common presenting symptom of nuchal or oropharyngeal teratomas is polyhydramnios and preterm labor.

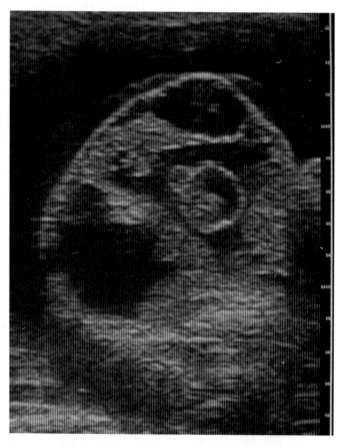

FIG. 10-23. This is a transverse view of a nuchal teratoma. The cervical spine is to the lower right of the image. The typical appearance of disorganized cystic and solid elements is seen. This infant presented with polyhydramnios and preterm labor and, despite all efforts, died after birth. (*Source:* Reprinted from Seeds JW, Azizkhan RG. *Congenital Malformations: Antenatal Diagnosis, Perinatal Management, and Counseling.* Rockville, MD: Aspen Publishers Inc, ©1990; p. 123.)

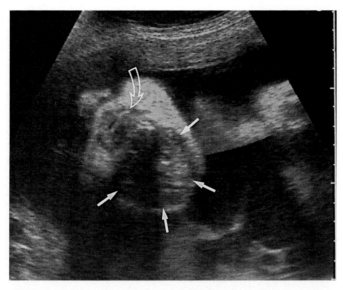

FIG. 10-24. The *small arrows* outline a soft-tissue mass beneath the fetal tongue. The *open arrow* indicates the fetal lips. This proved to be a teratoma. (*Source:* Reprinted from Seeds JW, Azizkhan RG. *Congenital Malformations: Antenatal Diagnosis, Perinatal Management, and Counseling.* Rockville, MD: Aspen Publishers Inc, ©1990; p. 124.)

Cystic Hygroma

A soft tissue mass arising from the occipital midline containing multiple internal fluid-filled compartments is likely a cystic hygroma (Fig. 10-25). These tumors may at times be difficult to distinguish from occipital encephaloceles. The compartments represent obstructed lymphatic channels. Aneuploidy is common in fetuses with a cystic hygroma, with about 6/10 45X Turner syndrome, and another 1/10 trisomy 21. The finding of a cystic hygroma along with fetal hydrops has an ominous prognosis even with a normal karyotype. Few survivors, if any, have been recorded from such a combination of findings.

Intracranial Tumors

Glioblastomas, teratomas, and craniopharyngiomas have been diagnosed antenatally and carry a poor but not absolute prognosis that depends on malignant potential, size, and resectability.

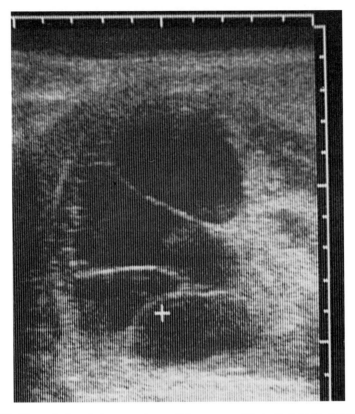

FIG. 10-25. The typical cystic hygroma is a soft-tissue mass filled with fluid-filled channels and septations as seen here. The fluid is lymph, and the channels are lymphatics. Often aneuploid, the prognosis is more severe if associated with hydrops.

SUMMARY

The ability of high-resolution realtime ultrasound to provide good quality images of the anatomy of the unborn is well known. The quality of the images may exceed the quality of the interpretation. The visualization of certain malformations does not imply certain knowledge of prognosis and therefore places a special burden on those who would counsel pregnancy management on the basis of such visualization. The dilemmas posed by this new technology include

1. Accuracy of diagnosis.
    What is the quality of images and interpretation?
2. Accuracy and precision of prognosis
    Do we really know the full meaning of what we see?
3. Quality of management counseling
    Are we really letting the patient decide?
    What should the patient's input be?

4. Adequacy of follow-up
   Are we facilitating or disabling grieving?
   Does the husband grieve?
   Does the couple understand recurrence risk?
   Is the couple aware of early diagnosis?

FURTHER READING

Chervenak FA, *et al*. The natural history of ventriculomegaly in a fetus without obstructive hydrocephalus. *Am J Obstet Gynecol* 1985;152:574.

Chervenak FA, *et al*. The management of fetal hydrocephalus. *Am J Obstet Gynecol* 1985;151:933.

Chervenak FA, *et al*. Diagnosis and management of fetal holoprosencephaly. *Obstet Gynecol* 1985;66: 322.

Chervenak FA, *et al*. Advances in the diagnosis of fetal defects. *N Engl J Med* 1986;315:305.

Clewell WH, *et al*. Ventriculomegaly: evaluation and management. *Semin Perinat* 1985;9:98.

Fiske CE, Filly RA. Ultrasound evaluation of the normal and abnormal fetal neural axis. *Radiol Clin North Am* 1982;20:285.

Greene MF, *et al*. Hydranencephaly: US appearance during in utero evolution. *Radiology* 1985;156:779.

Hirsch JF, *et al*. The Dandy-Walker malformation. *J Neurosurg* 1984;61:515.

Lipman SP, *et al*. Fetal intracranial teratoma: US diagnosis of three cases and a review of the literature. *Radiology* 1985;157:491.

McCullough DC, Balzer-Martin LA. Current prognosis in overt neonatal hydrocephalus. *J Neurosurg* 1982;57:378.

Pretorius D, *et al*. Clinical course of fetal hydrocephalus: 40 cases. *AJR* 1985;144:827.

Riboni G, *et al*. Ultrasound appearance of a glioblastoma in a 33-week fetus in utero. *J Clin Ultrasound* 1985;13:345.

Sawaya R, McLaurin RL. Dandy-Walker syndrome. *J Neurosurg* 1981;55:89.

Snyder JR, *et al*. Antenatal ultrasound diagnosis of an intracranial neoplasm. (craniopharyngioma). *J Clin Ultrasound* 1986;14:304.

11

Cardiothoracic Sonography

The fetal chest offers a unique challenge during the ultrasound examination. The bony rib cage, frequent interference by overlying limbs, rapid heart rate, and mobility of the fetus seem to conspire to hinder a careful examination of the heart, lungs, and mediastinum. At the same time, this part of the routine examination of the fetus is important in that congenital heart defects are the most common cause of neonatal deaths secondary to birth defects, are frequent components of the phenotypes of genetic and chromosomal disorders, and often occur in families with no known historic risk factors.

CHEST IMAGING

It is best to image the chest with the fetus in the spine-down position. If this is noted even early in the scan sequence, interrupt the usual format in order to take advantage of this fortuitous finding. Scan the fetal thorax in its entirety in both the transverse and sagittal planes. To develop ideal images of the soft tissue of the chest, align the transducer with the entire length of a rib and then slide the transducer slightly up or down to the intercostal space. Although this will not result in a perfectly transverse scanplane due to the slightly oblique nature of the normal rib alignment, it will afford a clear picture of the underlying soft tissue (Fig. 11-1). If the fetus maintains a spine-up position during the entire examination, one can usually get adequate images of the lungs and great vessels (although not usually of the heart) by scanning longitudinally parallel to the fetal spine and sliding the transducer from side to side in order to image the entire lung field (Fig. 11-2). If necessary, bring the patient back at a later time for re-examination.

In the normal fetus, the lungs are homogeneous in appearance and only slightly more echogenic than is the adjacent liver. A thin hypoechoic line may separate the liver from the lung. This line may not represent the true diaphragm as much as the interface between the two structures, and its presence alone is not satisfactory documentation of diaphragmatic integrity (Fig. 11-3A,B). Other than small, round vascular structures posterior to the heart near the midline, there should be no lung echolucencies.

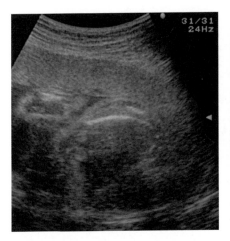 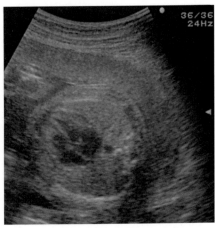

FIG. 11-1. The image on the left demonstrates the full length of a fetal rib in the leading hemithorax. By sliding the transducer parallel to this rib and imaging between ribs, a clear four-chamber view of the heart is obtained.

Intrathoracic pathology is unusual and is frequently heralded by either a mass effect with a shifted mediastinum, pleural effusions, or cystic or solid structures within the thorax. Table 11-1 lists the previously detected fetal chest masses. Evaluation of the fetus with hydrops or polyhydramnios should include a careful cardiothoracic examination: lesions that deviate the systemic venous return or obstruct the esophagus in the chest could reasonably produce these findings.

Characteristics to note about chest masses include their relative echodensity, presence of loculations, location in the chest, presence of mediastinal shift, and appearance of the contralateral chest if a unilateral lesion is found. Unfortunately,

TABLE 11-1. *Chest masses encountered by ultrasound in the fetus*

Diaphragmatic hernia
Congenital cystic adenomatoid malformations (CCAM)
Bronchogenic cysts
Pulmonary sequestrations: extralobar and intralobar
Neurenteric cysts
Anterior meningoceles
Mediastinal teratomas
Esophageal duplication cysts
Pleural effusions: isolated or as a component of hydrops

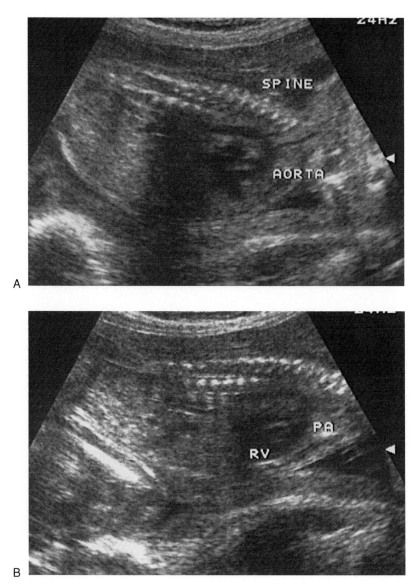

FIG. 11-2. The fetal spine might obscure a four-chamber view but it may be possible to obtain clear images of **(A)** the aortic arch with cephalic vessels seen arising from the arch and **(B)** the pulmonary arch. (*RV*, right ventricle; *PA*, pulmonary artery).

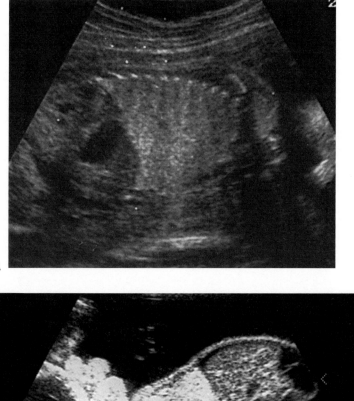

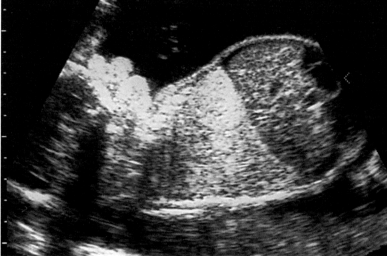

FIG. 11-3. A: The fetal lung should be slightly more echogenic than the liver. In this image, the stomach is the hypoechoic area in the abdomen. **B:** The abnormal contrast between the echogenicity of the lung and liver in this fetus is related to pulmonary lymphangiectasia. The differential diagnosis includes cystic adenomatoid malformation (CAM).

even in the presence of a unilateral lung lesion, significant contralateral pulmonary hypoplasia can occur if there is a mass effect. The status of the contralateral lung will influence prognosis. If a cystic mass or masses are noted in the fetal chest, careful attention to the position of the abdominal viscera should be made. While a normal position of the fetal stomach does not rule out a diaphragmatic hernia, it does diminish the odds (Figs. 11-4–11-6).

While it is uncommon, but relatively easy, to visualize a fetal chest mass, pulmonary hypoplasia presents a different dilemma. There is a spectrum of severity of pulmonary hypoplasia, and arguments about the best way to make the diagnosis on autopsy series emphasize the difficulty of a definitive diagnosis prenatally.

Normal lung development occurs from about 26 days post-conception throughout early childhood. Space-occupying lesions or longstanding oligohydramnios prior to alveolization can retard this process and result in lung development inadequate for postnatal lung function. While profound hypoplasia can sometimes be detected, milder forms cannot. Vintzeleos and others compared six different ultrasonographic methods for predicting lethal hypoplasia and found that the best measurement had only an 83% positive predictive value and an 85% negative predictive value. It must be remembered, therefore, that definitive prenatal diagnosis may not be possible (Figs. 11-7,11-8).

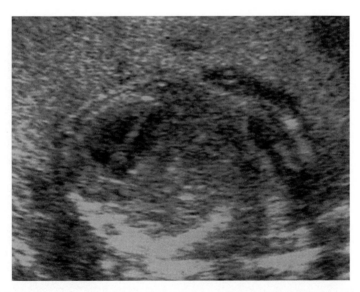

FIG. 11-4. This transverse view of the chest shows extreme deviation of the heart to the right hemithorax. Echogenic patches in the left hemithorax result from loops of small bowel in the chest through a large left-sided diaphragmatic hernia. The stomach has not herniated. Deviation of the heart is an important clue to the presence of chest masses.

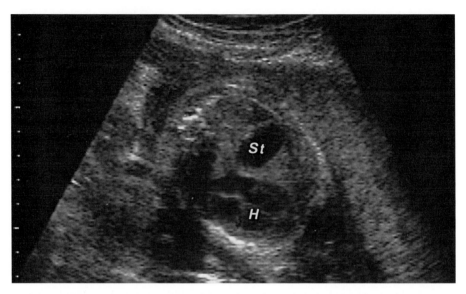

FIG. 11-5. The stomach *(St)* has herniated into the chest in this fetus with diaphragmatic hernia *(H)*. The heart is deviated to the right, and it is difficult to define the lung in either side of the chest.

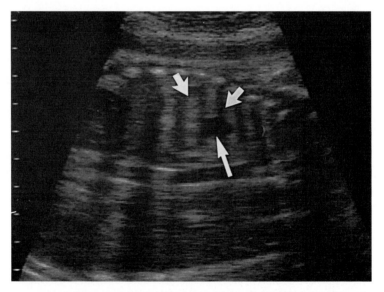

FIG. 11-6. A round hypoechoic mass is present in the left mid-lung field outlined by *arrows.* The remainder of the lung looks normal. The stomach is seen as a hypoechoic area in the abdomen. This was a pulmonary sequestration, but could have been a cystic adenomatoid malformation or bronchogenic cyst.

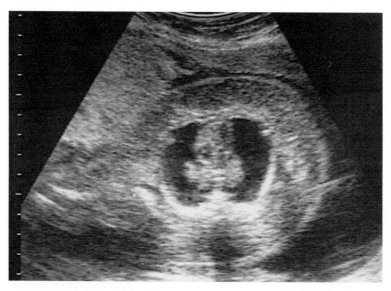

FIG. 11-7. Massive skin edema and pleural effusions are seen in this image from a fetus with nonimmune hydrops fetalis. Small, compressed lung buds on either side of the mediastinum make pulmonary hypoplasia a likely finding in this fetus.

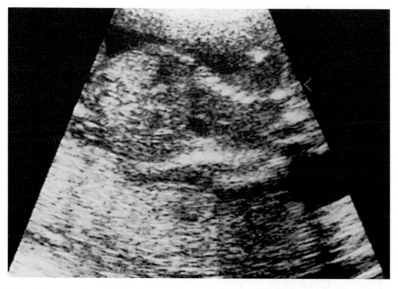

FIG. 11-8. Pulmonary hypoplasia is likely as a result of a skeletal dysplasia in this fetus. The thorax is constricted giving the appearance of a pear or bell-shaped body. The thoracic diameter should more closely approximate the abdominal diameter.

CARDIAC IMAGING

While intrinsic thoracic abnormalities are uncommon findings, cardiac anomalies are more common. The fetal cardiac examination is frequently the source of some concern for the sonographer because of the perceived difficulty of the study. The provider must be willing to practice this examination on every study done and to refer patients liberally if an abnormality is detected or until his or her ability to see normal anatomy is adequate.

Both the American Institute for Ultrasound in Medicine (AIUM) and the American College of Obstetrics & Gynecology (ACOG) include a four-chamber view of the fetal heart as part of the basic ultrasound examination because the majority of major congenital heart defects will alter the four-chamber view (Fig. 11-9). Thus, it is a reasonable screening method. On the other hand, for women with significant risk factors for fetal congenital heart disease, a diagnostic sonogram should be performed. This chapter will focus on the screening study and ultrasonic appearance of the great vessels.

The four-chamber view may be easily obtained in the spine-down fetus by imaging transversely at the level in the abdomen at which the abdominal circumference is measured. Angle the transducer cephalad to the fetus. That should produce a four-chamber view. Alternatively, align the transducer with the entire length of one of the lower ribs and then slide the transducer into the intercostal space, parallel to the rib. This likewise should produce a four-chamber image of the heart. Table 11-2 lists the components of the four-chamber view that must be

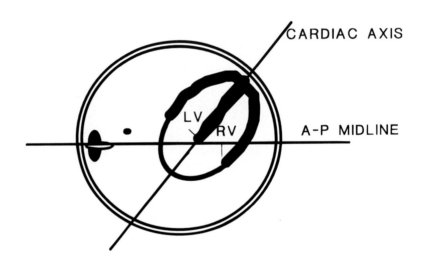

FOUR CHAMBER VIEW: FETAL HEART

FIG. 11-9. In a normal four-chamber view of the heart, an imaginary line drawn through the anterior/posterior midline will cross the right ventricle. The angle formed by this line and another drawn along the axis of the interventricular septum should approximate 45°.

TABLE 11–2. *Normal four-chamber heart view components*

Ventricular anatomy
  Both ventricles should be approximately equal in size.
  The moderator band may be visible within the cavity of the right ventricle.
  The interventricular septum should appear intact.
Atrial anatomy
  Both atria should be approximately equal in size.
  An echogenic line, (representing the foramen ovale) parallel to the interatrial septum should
    be seen moving into the left atrium.
  The interatrial septum should be interrupted in its central portion.
  The left atrium may have two or more irregular echolucencies arising from them, representing
    the pulmonary veins.
Atrioventricular valves
  The tricuspid valve should insert a very small distance down the interventricular septum toward
    the apex relative to the mitral valve.
Position
  An imaginary line drawn from the spine to the midline anterior chest wall should cross the
    right ventricle.
Size
  The heart should occupy no more than 50% of the area of chest image.
Rate
  The heart rate should be between 120 and 160 beats per minute and regular.

seen in order to document a normal study. In recent series of prenatally diagnosed congenital heart defects from tertiary centers, an abnormal screening ultrasound is the primary indication for referral (Fig. 11-10).

The four-chamber view is obtainable, according to Copel, in more than 95% of cases scanned between 18 weeks and term at a tertiary care center. This high

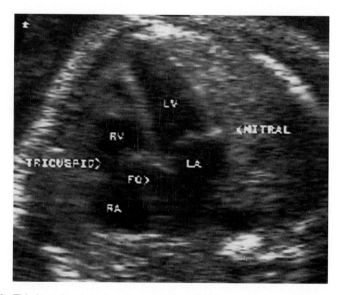

FIG. 11-10. This four chamber view demonstrates all of the components of a normal heart. *RV,* right ventricle; *LV,* left ventricle; *RA,* right atrium; *FO,* foramen ovale.

rate of observation of this particular view of the heart should not be significantly lower in an office-based practice after the initial skills are mastered. The ability to obtain the four-chamber view prior to 18 weeks is less predictable, mostly because of the small size of the heart, but it is possible, and it should be sought. By the same token, in the near-term fetus, it may be more difficult to image a four-chamber view because of a persistent spine-up position and the thickness of the fetal ribs and chest, which limit the acoustic window.

The four-chamber view, although a critical component of a basic fetal examination, is only a screening test. Many authors have documented defects that do not alter the four-chamber view. For instance, Bromly noted in a series of 69 fetuses with congenital heart defects scanned after 18 weeks that 63% were identified if only a four-chamber view were used, while 83% were identified if the great vessels were also imaged.

The aorta originates from the center of the heart from the left ventricle. The so-called five-chamber heart view that includes the aortic outflow tract is obtained from the four-chamber view by angling the transducer toward the right side of the heart and rotating it until the interventricular septum is seen in continuity with the medial wall of the aorta. In this view, the proximal aorta and aortic valve can be visualized and the mitral-aortic continuity area can be examined to assess the integrity of the left heart (Figs. 11-11,11-12).

To obtain an image of the pulmonary artery, angle the transducer from the five-chamber view cephalad and anterior to the fetus. The pulmonary artery can be seen in this manner with a surprisingly minute adjustment of the transducer

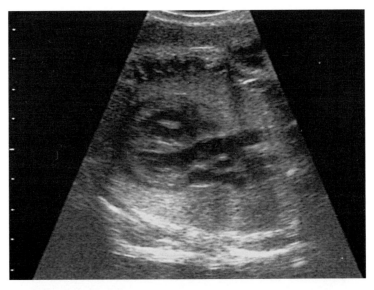

FIG. 11-11. The aorta is imaged here in this slightly oblique view of the fetal chest. The medial wall of the aorta is in continuity with the interventricular septum. The bright echo within the right ventricle is the moderator band.

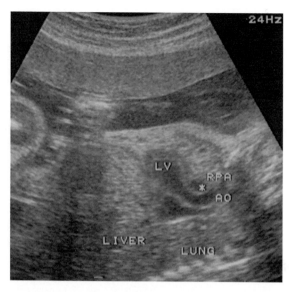

FIG. 11-12. In this sagittal image, the aorta *(AO)* is seen to arise from the left ventricle *(LV)*. The right pulmonary artery *(RPA)* is immediately anterior to the ascending aorta.

orientation as both great vessels arise from the medial sides of their respective ventricles (Fig. 11-13).

Normally, the aorta and pulmonary artery are approximately equal in caliber, although it is acceptable for the pulmonary artery to be 1–2 millimeters larger in transverse diameter measured at the level of the valve. The cross-over of the great

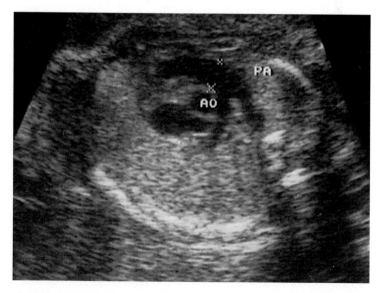

FIG. 11-13. Pulmonary artery is measured at about the level of the valve. Ductus arteriosus and right pulmonary artery are seen at the level of their bifurcation, with the aorta posterior.

vessels, with a nonparallel orientation of the outflow tracts helps rule out major anomalies of the conotruncus.

In order to confirm that there is a normal orientation of the vessels to the ventricles, that is, that there is no transposition of the great vessels, a long-axis view is obtained. In this view, visible usually when the fetus is either spine-up or -down, is obtained longitudinally and parasagittally. The aorta tightly curves from the heart center, arches, and then forms the descending aorta. One must confirm the presence of the cephalic vessels arising from this candy-cane-shaped vessel to be certain that it is the aorta. The pulmonary artery arises anteriorly, takes a wider sweep posteriorly than the aorta in a hockey-stick-shaped curve to connect via the ductal arch to the aorta. The trifurcation of the main pulmonary artery to form the ductus arteriosus and right and left pulmonary artery without cephalic vessels confirms its identification.

Some defects are impossible to exclude by prenatal sonography. Due to the normal presence of the foramen ovale and ductus arteriosus, minor abnormalities of the interatrial septum or persistent patent ductus cannot be excluded. In addition, the interventricular septum is a nonplanar three-dimensional structure and cannot be visualized in its entirety. Therefore, small ventricular septal defects cannot be excluded. Ventricular septal defects (VSDs) are important findings, however, as they are the most common congenital heart defects and are frequently seen as a component of more complex congenital heart disease. The prenatal diagnosis of a VSD is not only difficult to exclude for reasons noted above, but also difficult to confirm. Many small VSDs may close spontaneously *in utero,* so they may not be confirmed by postnatal examination. In addition, if the examination is done with the septum parallel to the scan beam, there can be significant signal drop out, especially at the crux of the heart, mimicking a subvalvular VSD (Fig. 11-14). For this reason, a suspected VSD should be visualized in two scanplanes at the same examination to make the diagnosis. Importantly, some heart lesions are flow dependent. For instance, hypoplasia of one of the ventricles may result from a primary valvular lesion that limits blood flow into the ventricle. Over time with an abnormally low blood flow, the ventricle may become hypoplastic.

These caveats emphasize the importance of appropriate referral for diagnostic echocardiography versus performing an adequate screening study such as one would for all scanned patients. Table 11-3 lists the standard recommendations for echocardiographic referral. Components of a full echocardiographic examination may include a more detailed examination of the anatomy of the intracardiac and extracardiac anatomy, M-mode studies to assess contractility and rhythm, pulsed Doppler documentation of flow and color Doppler assessment of flow patterns. It is important to recognize that the same difficulties with fetal size and position will challenge the echocardiographer, and repeat studies may be needed.

The goals of this chapter have been primarily to introduce the sonographer to principles of cardiothoracic sonography and to emphasize normal findings. As stated earlier, however, the majority of cases of congenital heart disease occurs among fetuses at low risk for such problems. Consequently, the remainder of this

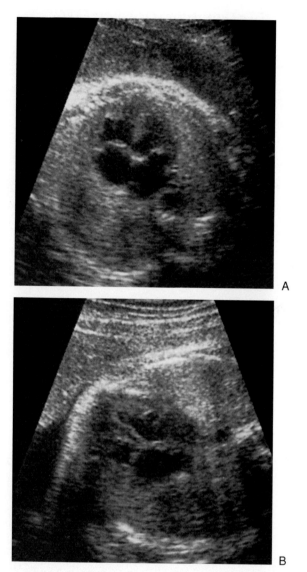

A

B

FIG. 11-14. Two images of the same fetus obtained from different angles. **A:** the interventricular septum is nearly parallel to the ultrasound beam. This produces an image suspicious for a subvalvular VSD. By imaging the septum at a different angle more perpendicular to the beam, the septum appears intact **(B)**.

TABLE 11–3. *Recommendations for referral for fetal echocardiography*

1. Abnormal screening ultrasound
2. Known fetal aneuploidy
3. Maternal diabetes
4. Family history of congenital heart disease
5. Presence of extracardiac malformations, including hydrops
6. Maternal phenylketonuria or oral accutane use in the first trimester
7. Maternal alcohol abuse
8. Persistent fetal arrhythmia

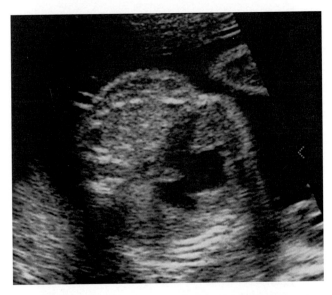

FIG. 11-15. The ventricles here are asymmetric. The interventricular septum is wedge shaped and ends prematurely producing a large interventricular septal defect. The thickened tissue between the right atrium and right ventricle is a common atrioventricular valve.

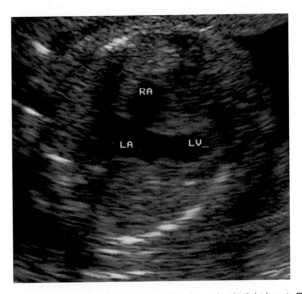

FIG. 11-16. No right ventricle is seen in this fetus with a hypoplastic right heart. *RA*, right atrium; *LA*, left atrium; *LV*, left ventricle.

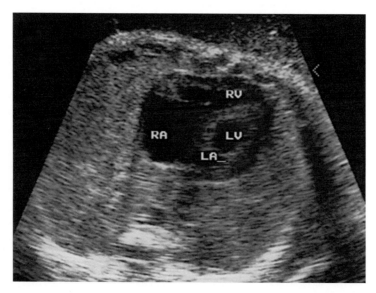

FIG. 11-17. The left ventricular wall is hypertrophied and the chamber of the left ventricle *(LV)* is small, as is the left atrium *(LA)*. With hypoplastic left heart, the right sided structures may enlarge in order to handle the entire cardiac output, as is shown here. *RA,* right atrium; *RV,* right ventricle.

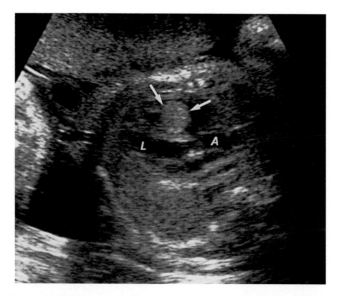

FIG. 11-18. A round, echodense tumor *(arrows)* arises from the right side of the interventricular septum. Rhabdomyomas may be solitary or multiple and may appear in any location in the heart. *A,* atrium; *L,* lung.

TABLE 11–4. *Abnormalities detectable by alterations in the four-chamber view*

Asymmetry of atria
  Right larger than left
    Tricuspid valve atresia or stenosis
    Pulmonary valve atresia or stenosis
    Coarctation of the aorta
    Anomalous pulmonary venous drainage
    Hypoplastic left heart
    Ebstein's anomaly
    Uteroplacental insufficiency
  Left larger than right
    Mitral valve atresia or stenosis
    Aortic valve atresia or stenosis
    Hypoplastic right heart

Asymmetry of the ventricles
  Right larger than left
    Pulmonary valve atresia or stenosis
    Coarctation of the aorta
    Hypoplastic left heart
    Anomalous pulmonary venous drainage
  Left larger than right
    Aortic valve stenosis or atresia
    Hypoplastic right heart

Abnormal axis
  Any disorder involving the conotruncus
  Mass lesions in the chest

Disruption of cardiac tissue
  Abnormal valve development
  Large ventricular septal defects
  Large atrial septal defects
  Rhabdomyoma

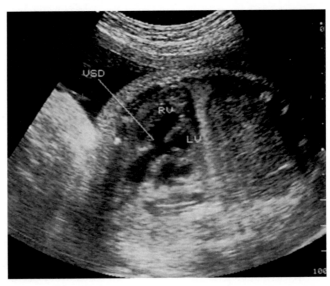

FIG. 11-19. A large VSD is noted with an outflow tract sitting astride the interventricular septum. This fetus has double outlet right ventricle, but tetrology of Fallot would have been possible.

chapter includes photos and a table illustrating common malformations that you might see on 2D echo (Table 11-4; Figures 11-15–11-19).

FURTHER READING

Albright EB, Crane JP, Shackelford GD. Prenatal diagnosis of a bronchogenic cyst. *J Ultrasound Med* 1988;7:91–5.

Callan NA, Maggio M, Steger S, Kan JS. Fetal echocardiography: indications for referral, prenatal diagnosis, and outcomes. *Am J Perinatol* 1991;8:390–4.

Copel JA, Pilu G, Green J, Hobbins JC, Kleinman CS. Fetal echocardiographic screening for congenital heart disease: the importance of the four-chamber view. *Am J Obstet Gynecol* 1987;157:648–55.

Hegge FN, Lees MH, Watson PT. Utility of a screening examination the fetal cardiac position and four chambers during obstetric sonography. *J Reprod Med* 1987;32:353–8.

Reece EA, Lockwood CJ, Rizzo N, Pilu G, Bovicelli L, Hobbins JC. Intrinsic intrathoracic malformations of the fetus: sonographic detection and clinical presentation. *Obstet Gynecol* 1987;75:627–32.

Sadler, TW. *Langman's Medical Embryology,* 6th ed. Baltimore: Williams & Wilkins. 1990;228–36.

Smith RS, Comstock CH, Kirk JS, Lee W. Ultrasonographic left cardiac axis deviation: a marker for fetal anomalies. *Obstet Gynecol* 1995;85(2):187–91.

Vergani P, Mariani S, Ghidini A, Schiavina R, Cavallone M, Locatelli A, *et al.* Screening for congenital heart disease with the four chamber view of the fetal heart. *Am J Obstet Gynecol* 1992:167:1000–3.

Vintzileos AM, Campbell WA, Rodis JF, Nochimson DJ, Pinette MG, Petrikovsky BM. Comparison of six different ultrasonographic methods for predicting lethal fetal pulmonary hypoplasia. *Am J Obstet Gynecol* 1989;161:606–12.

12

Sonographic Evaluation of Fetal Abdominal and Renal Malformations

The sonographic evaluation of the fetal abdomen and urinary tract requires not only the direct visual assessment of anatomy but often the parallel evaluation of features of functionally related abnormalities. These include oligo- or polyhydramnios, abdominal circumference, and the heart-to-chest ratio that might be altered in the case of pulmonary hypoplasia. Structural abnormalities of the abdominal wall, gastrointestinal abnormalities, and urinary tract abnormalities may all be detected with ultrasound, but diagnosis is likely only if the examiner methodically evaluates key features of anatomy.

FETAL ABDOMINAL SCREENING: NORMAL ANATOMY

Sonographic screening of the fetal abdomen in the low-risk pregnancy may be accomplished with two transverse views that document a normal-size, fluid-filled fetal stomach in the left upper quadrant and a normal umbilical insertion in the lower anterior midline. In the first view (Fig. 12-1), the liver normally occupies about 60% of the area of the trunk section at the level of the stomach and is relatively homogeneous in echotexture. The umbilical vein is in the anteroposterior (AP) midline opposite the spine, while the gall bladder is to the right side of the midline. There is normally no free peritoneal fluid seen. At the level of the umbilical insertion (Fig. 12-2), the kidneys are typically lateral to the spine in the dorsal abdomen (Fig. 12-3). The renal pelves may or may not be discretely seen within the mid-kidney, measuring no more than 5–6 mm in anteroposterior (AP) diameter in the normal case (Fig. 12-4). The umbilical insertion itself is typically an abrupt attachment of the cord, with the vessels seen to enter through the abdominal wall. The intestinal structures in early gestation are vague and show lit-

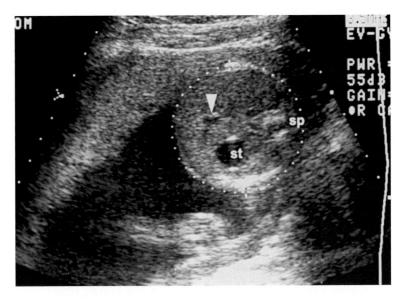

FIG. 12-1. This transverse upper abdominal view demonstrates the fetal spine *(sp)*, the fetal stomach *(st)*, and the umbilical vein within the liver mass *(arrowhead)*. The abdominal circumference is being measured. The kidneys may be seen as slightly echospared, circular areas on either side of the spine.

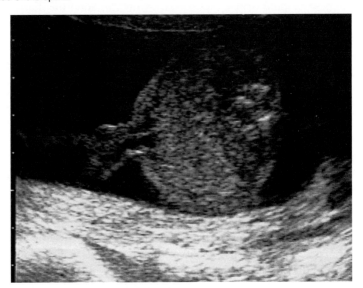

FIG. 12-2. Sliding the transducer a bit caudally from Fig. 12-1, the umbilical insertion is seen opposite the spine in the sagittal midline. Again, the kidneys are seen as vague echospared areas on either side of the spine. (*Source:* Reprinted from Seeds JW, Azizkhan RG. *Congenital Malformations: Antenatal Diagnosis, Perinatal Management, and Counseling.* Aspen Publishers, Inc. © 1990; p. 298.)

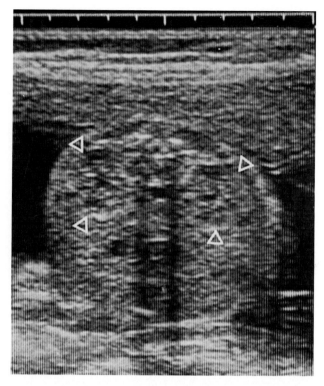

FIG. 12-3. In early gestation, the kidneys are not readily apparent. In this view, the kidneys are highlighted by *open triangles* on either side of the spinal shadow.

tle anatomic organization visually, but, later in gestation, the large intestine may demonstrate discrete definition as it fills with mature meconium (Fig. 12-5). The small intestine is not seen as a discretely outlined organ at any time in normal pregnancy. The bladder is a discretely outlined symmetrical anechoic structure in the low anterior midline of the pelvis and abdomen.

The abdominal circumference (AC) bears a moderately close relationship to gestational age and may be useful for estimation of fetal weight. AC may be abnormally large for gestational age in the case of macrosomia, fetal ascites, large urinary tract masses, or fetal bowel obstruction, but typically small for gestational age in the case of esophageal obstruction, gastroschisis, or intrauterine growth restriction (IUGR) from other causes.

Abdominal Malformations

Abdominal malformations other than urinary tract fall into several categories including:

      ventral wall defects
      bowel obstruction
      ascites
      mass lesions

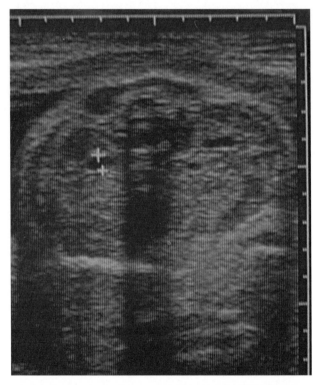

FIG. 12-4. The renal pelves are sometimes seen as here, but the A-P measurement should not exceed 4 mm up to 20 weeks, 7 mm from 20–30 weeks, and 10 mm past 30 weeks. If renal pyelectasis exceeds these standards, serial monitoring is recommended and neonatal study to identify correctable abnormalities. (*Source:* Reprinted from Seeds JW, Azizkhan RG. *Congenital Malformations: Antenatal Diagnosis, Perinatal Management, and Counseling.* Aspen Publishers, Inc. © 1990; p. 340.)

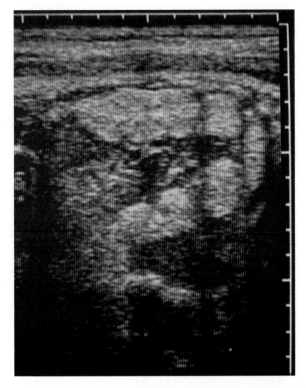

FIG. 12-5. Near term, the mature fetal bowel filled with meconium may present this echogenic appearance without the implication of pathology.

VENTRAL WALL DEFECTS

Omphalocele

By the end of the eighth week after conception (10th week menstrual), the leaflets of the fetal abdominal wall should have merged at the umbilicus forming the umbilical annulus, and the abdominal viscera become enclosed within the coelomic cavity. In about 30% of cases, a "physiologic" omphalocele may remain at 11 weeks (Fig. 12-6), but by 12 weeks postmenstrual, the umbilicus is normally completed.

If the process of visceral return to the coelomic cavity remains incomplete beyond the 12th week, various organs will continue to grow and develop within the proximal umbilical cord. This produces a soft tissue mass anterior to the lower midline fetal abdomen covered by a thin but distinct membrane that constitutes an **omphalocele** (Fig. 12-7). The covering membrane is composed of peritoneum

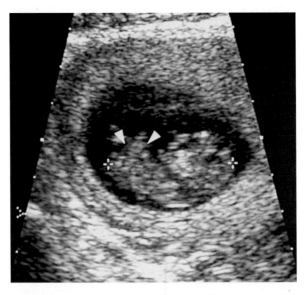

FIG. 12-6. By 11 weeks gestation, the majority of fetuses will have a normal umbilical insertion, but 30% will demonstrate a "physiologic omphalocele" *(arrowheads)*. By 12 weeks, all normal fetal umbilical insertions appear as expected, with all viscera within the abdominal cavity.

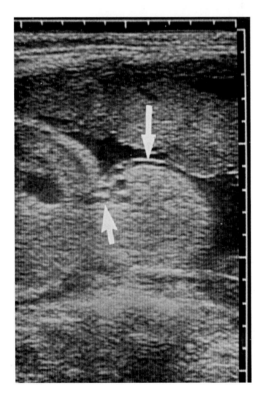

FIG. 12-7. An omphalocele is best seen in a transverse view at the level of the umbilicus. The soft tissue mass replaces the umbilicus, and the tissues are covered by a bilayer membrane. The umbilical vessels are seen to traverse the soft tissue mass, and the cord should be found to insert on the mass.

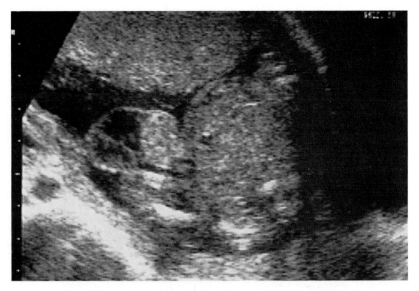

FIG. 12-8. Exclusion of omphalocele requires careful examination of the insertion site. This cord insertion demonstrates a very small omphalocele that carries at least the same implications for aneuploidy and associated malformations as the larger types.

and amnion. The omphalocele mass may be small (Fig. 12-8) or large. The umbilical cord inserts on the omphalocele, and the vessels are seen to enter the fetal trunk from the mass. There is a high association between omphalocele and aneuploidy (30–50%), and there is a high association with significant other malformations (40–70%). In the absence of aneuploidy or another malformation that independently compromises survival, survival after successful repair is reported to be 95%.

Obstetrical management has been the topic of some controversy over the past decade, with few observers able to produce hard data supporting a benefit from arbitrary cesarean delivery. However, in the case of a large omphalocele, scheduled atraumatic delivery in a center prepared for the special needs of such an infant clearly contributes to a good outcome.

Gastroschisis

Either as a result of a vascular occlusion or faulty involution of an umbilical vein in early embryogenesis, a through-and-through defect in the fetal abdomi-

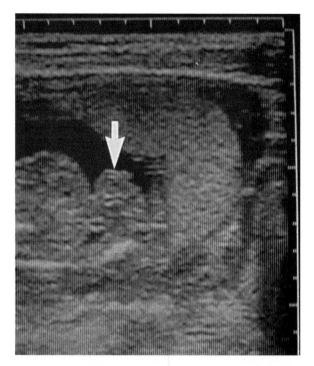

FIG. 12-9. Gastroschisis in the early fetus is shown here at 18 weeks. In the early fetus, the bowel may present a reasonably unified appearance and may be difficult to confidently discriminate from omphalocele. Absence of a covering membrane and location of the cord insertion adjacent to the origin of the herniated bowel should alert the examiner.

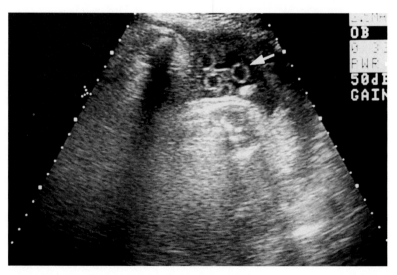

FIG. 12-10. Later in gestation, the bowel loops may separate and be seen distinct from one another. After 26 weeks, increased osmolarity of the amniotic fluid produces a subserosal inflammation and sonographic thickening of the bowel wall as shown here *(arrow)*.

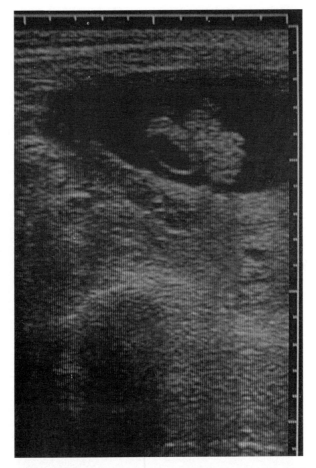

FIG. 12-11. Body stalk malformation produces extreme dorsiflexion of the fetal spine, and free floating viscera as demonstrated here.

nal wall just above and to the right of the umbilicus results in the herniation of various amounts of small bowel into the amniotic cavity an is called **gastroschisis.** Early in gestation, the sonographic appearance of gastroschisis bears some resemblance to omphalocele (Fig. 12-9), but, later, the thickened echogenic walls of the small bowel often develop a subserosal inflammatory reaction to amniotic fluid, and this produces a characteristic appearance (Fig. 12-10). Aneuploidy is not more frequent in the case of gastroschisis, and other major malformations are much less frequent than with omphalocele. Survival and repairability here, too, are about 95%.

No conclusive evidence supports abdominal delivery, but a variety of observers have reported lower rates of necrotizing enterocolitis, shorter recovery times, and shorter neonatal intensive care days when abdominal delivery has been employed. Scheduled delivery with careful coordination of neonatal medical and surgical care is again an important part of a successful outcome.

Major Abdominal Wall Failure

Body Stalk Malformation

Occasionally, a fetus is encountered with apparent total failure of abdominal wall formation. All abdominal viscera are seen floating in the amniotic cavity

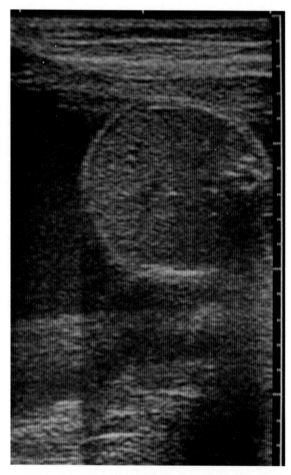

FIG. 12-12. The clinical combination of polyhydramnios, preterm labor, and a transverse abdominal view without stomach strongly suggests esophageal atresia. The large majority of esophageal atresias also have a tracheoesophageal fistula, though, and some fluid may be found in the stomach. Esophageal atresia carries up to a 30% risk of Down syndrome.

(Fig. 12-11), and sharp dorsiflexion of the fetal spine is often noted. The fetus is seen attached to the placenta and there is virtual absence of a true umbilical cord. The etiology of this rare but lethal malformation is obscure.

BOWEL OBSTRUCTION

Esophagus

The classic combination of polyhydramnios and absence of visualization of the fetal stomach despite repeated attempts is very suggestive but not diagnostic of esophageal obstruction (Fig. 12-12). The frequent (90%) association of a tracheoesophageal fistula with esophageal atresia often results in a visible stomach. Perhaps just as often, for reasons that are unclear, a normal fetus with polyhydramnios will be seen with a nonvisualized stomach. In the case of polyhydramnios and a nonvisualized stomach, repeat examinations over time is recommended with semiquantitative assessment of amniotic fluid. If the polyhydramnios is nonpathologic, the stomach will be seen in subsequent examinations, and the amniotic fluid excess is typically not progressive. If, however, esophageal obstruction is present, the amniotic fluid excess is most often seen to be progressive over time. Uterine fundal height should also be followed closely, as a secondary measure of fluid excess. If esophageal atresia is suspected, fetal aneuploidy must also be considered.

Duodenum

Polyhydramnios seen with double upper abdominal anechoic masses is very strong evidence for duodenal obstruction. The anechoic masses represent the stomach, narrowing to the pylorus, and the dilated duodenum proximal to the obstruction (Fig. 12-13). The AP midline should run between the two anechoic masses. The obstruction may be atresia, intraluminal webs, or an annular pancreas, but the neonatal implications are similar. These are almost always repairable, but there is 30% association between duodenal obstruction and Down syndrome. As with esophageal obstruction, the polyhydramnios will typically worsen over time, while idiopathic polyhydramnios more often remains stable.

Jejunum/Ileum

Polyhydramnios with a more linear, serpentine fluid-filled mass of the fetal abdomen is indicative of small bowel atresia or obstruction below the duodenum (Fig. 12-14). These are most often repairable but also carry an increased risk of fetal aneuploidy.

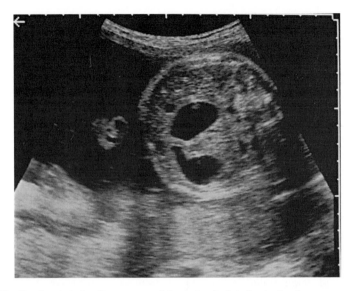

FIG. 12-13. Duodenal obstruction may result from atresia, intraluminal webs, or an annular pancreas. All produce the typical picture shown here. Transverse upper abdominal scans will show dual anechoic masses on either side of the midline representing dilated stomach narrowing to the piloris, then dilated duodenum proximal to the obstruction. All carry up to a 30% risk of Down syndrome. (*Source:* Reprinted from Seeds JW, Azizkhan RG. *Congenital Malformations: Antenatal Diagnosis, Perinatal Management, and Counseling.* Aspen Publishers, Inc. © 1990; p. 249.)

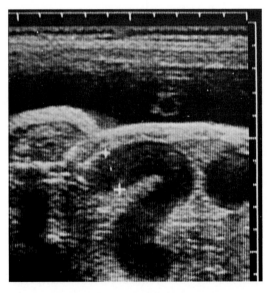

FIG. 12-14. Jejunal atresia results in a more serpentine fluid-filled abdominal mass as seen here. Typically, the contents of the small bowel are liquid and, therefore, relatively anechoic.

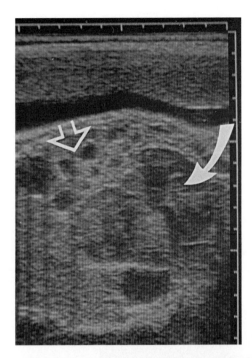

FIG. 12-15. A: Rupture of the large intestine, associated with a meconium ileus, produces an irregular mass *(curved arrow)* of mixed echotexture, with hyperparastaltic small bowel *(open arrow)*. There is a high association with cystic fibrosis. (*Source:* Reprinted from Seeds JW, Azizkhan RG. *Congenital Malformations: Antenatal Diagnosis, Perinatal Management, and Counseling.* Aspen Publishers, Inc. © 1990; p. 253.)

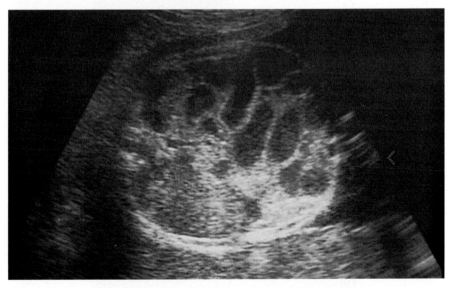

FIG. 12-15. B: This transverse abdominal view of a fetus that proved to have cystic fibrosis shows dilated and hyperparastaltic loops of small intestine associated with a meconium ileus.

Large Bowel/Meconium Peritonitis

Meconium ileus, and *in utero* volvulus with perforation will present a similar combination of polyhydramnios and a large, irregular, indistinct abdominal mass often with both fluid and soft tissue textures (Fig. 12-15A). There may be small bowel hyperperistalsis (Fig. 12-15B). In the case of meconium ileus, there is a 50% risk of cystic fibrosis.

Ascites

Hydrops fetalis is defined as fetal skin edema plus effusions in two of three serous cavities including the peritoneal, pleural, or pericardial cavities (Fig. 12-16). The relative proportions of these findings can vary, and, in occasional cases, the ascites can be the only real abnormality seen. Fetal ascites can result from severe hemolytic anemia or be a part of a variety of nonimmune causes that generally have portal hypertension in common. True ascites must be differentiated

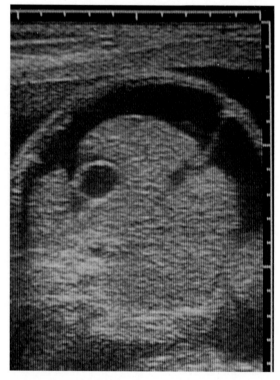

FIG. 12-16. The dark (anechoic) areas within this fetal abdomen represent fetal ascites. At about one o'clock is the falciform ligament extending from the fetal liver to the abdominal wall. To the left side of the liver is the stomach.

from the normal peritoneal echo drop out called *pseudoascites* by some authors. Furthermore, fetal ascites has been documented in more than one case to be transient followed by a good perinatal outcome. It is therefore impossible to accurately predict outcome in the case of isolated fetal ascites.

Other Masses

A variety of other fetal abdominal masses have been reported including ovarian cysts, liver hamartomas, omental cysts, and fetal hemangiomas. Often these are detected as the result of an examination done for dating purposes or as the result of the secondary polyhydramnios. Insufficient experience is yet accumulated in most cases to be able to accurately predict clinical outcome in the majority of these masses. The diagnosis of such a mass, therefore, is rarely the appropriate basis for pregnancy management decisions.

OBSTETRICAL MANAGEMENT AND ABDOMINAL MALFORMATIONS

Obstetrical management counseling consists of assessing the benefit of fetal karyotyping, assessment of fetal survival with or without disabilities, serial observation for appropriate growth and development, and choosing the appropriate method for delivery. In the case of omphalocele, esophageal, duodenal, and other small bowel obstruction, and ascites, fetal aneuploidy is sufficiently likely to suggest the benefit of fetal karyotyping. In the absence of other major malformations and in the absence of fetal aneuploidy, repair with survival without high probability of enduring disabilities is expected.

Gastroschisis carries no increased risk of aneuploidy and a high probability of survival without residua.

Body stalk abnormalities remain a fetal condition not associated with neonatal survival.

All of the above malformations benefit from referral and delivery by whatever means at a center prepared for and capable of the special care and surgical interventions required. Remote delivery and neonatal transport are not recommended as they are associated with a lower rate of successful long-term outcome.

FETAL RENAL MALFORMATIONS

The fetal urinary tract lends itself to sonographic diagnosis perhaps more than any other organ system. The sonographic visual contrast between anechoic fluid and echogenic tissue provides this level of diagnostic sensitivity. Amniotic fluid is virtually completely dependent on fetal urine output after 20 weeks gestation. If there is not a patent, functional urinary tract, there will be no amniotic fluid after 20 weeks.

The sonographic examination of the fetal urinary tract requires an assessment of each of the components individually and as a system. The kidneys, the bladder, and the amniotic fluid are connected. A serious problem with kidneys is unlikely if bladder filling and amniotic fluid volume appear normal. Likewise, a serious problem with the bladder is unlikely if the kidneys and amniotic fluid volume appear normal.

The fetal urinary tract should be part of every obstetrical ultrasound examination survey of fetal anatomy and includes the kidneys, the bladder, and the amniotic fluid.

Normal Sonographic Anatomy

The fetal kidneys are seen as symmetrical sonolucent soft tissue structures on either side of fetal spine in midtransverse scan of abdomen (Fig. 12-17). Normal longitudinal and AP dimensions are reported, and the normal kidney-to-abdominal circumference ratio is about .27–.31 from 24- to 36-weeks gestation.

The kidneys are not sharply outlined prior to 28 weeks, but perirenal fat highlights outline in third trimester. Renal pelvis is often not discretely seen but may

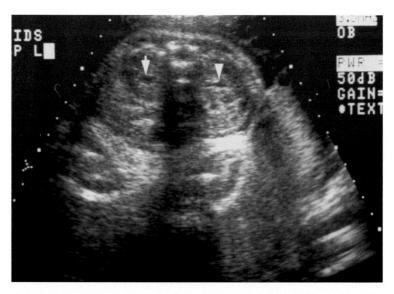

FIG. 12-17. Transverse *(left)* and longitudinal *(right)* views of the third trimester fetal kidneys demonstrate the echogenic outlines produced by perinephric fat laid down in the third trimester.

appear normally as anechoic area of midkidney, with AP diameter not more than 5 mm, or 50% of AP diameter of kidney in same plane.

The ureters are normally not visible.

The bladder is usually seen from 16 weeks gestation as anechoic area in mid-fetal pelvis seen to fill and empty on about an hourly cycle with typical dimensions of $14 \times 14 \times 25$ mm when full at 19 weeks, with capacity of about 5 cc.

Amniotic fluid is a physiologic extension of fetal urinary tract after 20 weeks. Prior to 18 weeks, fetal urine is not required, and 18–20 weeks is a transition period.

Malformation

Malformation of the fetal urinary tract may take one of four forms including agenesis, dysplasia, obstructive uropathy, or congenital nephrosis. Agenesis may be unilateral or bilateral, dysplasia may be polycystic or multicystic, and obstructive uropathy may involve the ureteropelvic junction, the ureterovessicle junction, or the urethra. Urethral obstruction may result from urethral valves, urethral atresia, or cloacal plate malformation. Certain of these malformations result effectively in no urine output, either no bladder filling or no bladder emptying, and severe oligohydramnios after 20 weeks. Pulmonary hypoplasia results from prolonged, severe oligohydramnios, and neonatal death occurs promptly from respiratory failure. If normal bladder filling and emptying and normal amniotic fluid volume is noted, pulmonary development and neonatal survival may be expected.

Renal Agenesis

Failure of renal development affects 0.1–.3 per 1000 live births, shows a male predominance, and a 2–4% recurrence risk. Severe oligohydramnios after 20 weeks (Fig. 12-18) is expected, and pulmonary hypoplasia is the rule. There are the typical compression deformities including brachycephaly, flattening of the face, and arthrogryposis of the large joints (Potter's syndrome) (Table 12-1). At sonography, the kidneys are not identified, there is no bladder filling, and severe oligohydramnios is seen. Adrenal hyperplasia is common, and occasionally the

TABLE 12–1. *Renal dysplasia: Potter classification*

Type I:	Infantile polycystic
Type II:	Congenital multicystic
Type III:	Adult polycystic
Type IV:	Secondary cystic dysplastic

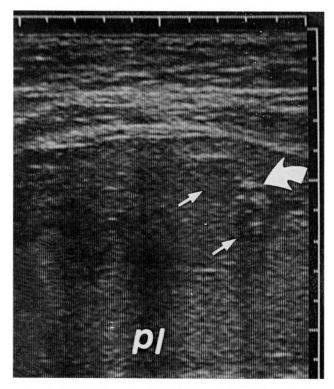

FIG. 12-18. Renal agenesis results in anhydramnios by 20 weeks gestation, elevated maternal serum alphafetoprotein, and, eventually, fetal pulmonary hypoplasia and neonatal death. The *large arrow* indicates the spine, the *small arrows* indicate hypertrophied adrenal glands occasionally mistaken for kidneys. Absence of amniotic fluid and bladder filling over time supports the diagnosis. pl, placenta. (*Source:* Reprinted from Seeds JW, Azizkhan RG. *Congenital Malformations: Antenatal Diagnosis, Perinatal Management, and Counseling.* Aspen Publishers, Inc. © 1990; p. 238.)

TABLE 12–2. *Comparison of polycystic and multicystic dysplasia*

	Polycystic	Multicystic
Incidence	1/5	4/5
Appearance	Echodense	Large cysts
Bilaterality	100%	20%
Survival	Rare	Expected
Recurrence	25%	3–5%

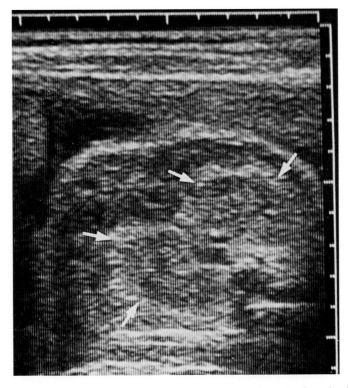

FIG. 12-19. Polycystic renal dysplasia produces many microscopic cysts of proximal collecting tubules and results in enlarged echogenic kidneys as shown here. The *small arrows* indicate the outlines of the kidneys. An autosomal recessive condition, oligohydramnios and pulmonary hypoplasia are expected but not absolute. (*Source:* Reprinted from Seeds JW, Azizkhan RG. *Congenital Malformations: Antenatal Diagnosis, Perinatal Management, and Counseling.* Aspen Publishers, Inc. © 1990; p. 331.)

adrenal glands mimic kidneys on the transverse view, but absent bladder filling and anhydramnios should be convincing evidence of agenesis.

Polycystic Dysplasia

Infantile polycystic dysplasia results in obstruction of the proximal collecting system and replacement of the kidneys with innumerable 1–2 mm cysts (Fig. 12-19). The sonographic result is enlarged, echodense kidneys, little or no bladder filling, and eventual anhydramnios in most cases. In the typical case, pulmonary hypoplasia leads to neonatal death. This condition affects 0.5 per 1000 live births. Occasional examples of incomplete expression, with preservation of small areas

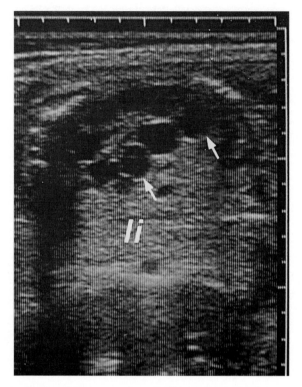

FIG. 12-20. Multicystic dysplasia is the more common type, is predominantly unilateral, and results from obstruction more distal in the collecting system. The visual result is a kidney replaced with many large macroscopic cysts *(arrows)*. Contralateral function is typically normal, bladder filling is normal, and lung development is not typically impaired. li, liver.

of normal renal tissue show urine production, bladder filling, and some maintenance of amniotic fluid. Therefore, complete exclusion with early ultrasound is not possible. Infantile polycystic dysplasia demonstrates an autosomal recessive pattern of inheritance, with a 25% risk of recurrence in a sibship (Table 12-2).

Multicystic Dysplasia

The more common dysplastic condition found is multicystic dysplasia, occurring in 2–3 per 1000 live births. Obstruction of a more distal portion of the collecting system results in relatively fewer, larger anechoic masses replacing the kidney (Fig. 12-20). Since multicystic dysplasia is unilateral 80% of the time, normal contralateral function results in normal bladder filling, normal amniotic

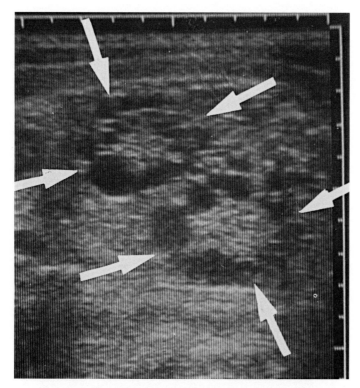

FIG. 12-21. About one in five cases of multicystic dysplasia is bilateral *(arrows)* as shown here, or rarely associated with contralateral agenesis. In either case, the result is no bladder filling, no amniotic fluid, pulmonary hypoplasia, and neonatal death.

fluid volume, lung development, and survival. If observed early in gestation, the cysts are typically seen to grow with time. Multicystic renal dysplasia follows a multifactorial, polygenic pattern of inheritance, with a 2–4% recurrence risk.

In the less common case of bilateral multicystic dysplasia (Fig. 12-21), or in combination with contralateral agenesis, absent urine production, absent bladder filling, absent amniotic fluid, and neonatal death are expected (Table 12-2).

OBSTRUCTIVE UROPATHY

Ureteropelvic Junction

Fetal pyelectasis is a common observation that may be benign or may result from ureteropelvic junction (UPJ) obstruction. The obstruction may be partial or complete, and the pyelectasis may be progressive or not. Typically unilateral obstruction often results in the progressive growth of the dilated renal pelvis (Fig. 12-22A,B), or the growth of a related retroperitoneal, perirenal urinoma (Fig. 12-23). Occasionally, a mass effect of the dilated pelvis or urinoma results in polyhydramnios and antenatal drainage, or treatment may be considered. Otherwise, antenatal treatment of the unilateral condition is not recommended.

Urethral Obstruction

Urethral obstruction may result from atresia, valves, or cloacal plate abnormality. The prognosis is somewhat different, and the possibility of benefit from antenatal treatment differs among these etiologies.

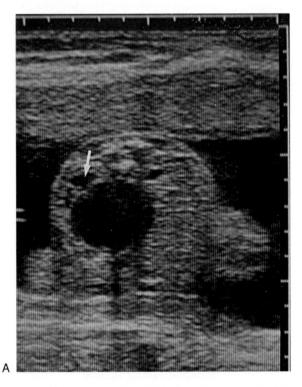

A

FIG. 12-22. A: Severe ureteropelvic junction obstruction produces severe intra- and extrarenal pyelectasis with caliectasis as shown here. The *arrow* indicates a dilated calix. The expansion of the renal pelvis may cause bowel displacement and dysfunction leading to polyhydramnios. (*Source:* Reprinted from Seeds JW, Azizkhan RG. *Congenital Malformations: Antenatal Diagnosis, Perinatal Management, and Counseling.* Aspen Publishers, Inc. © 1990; p. 341.)

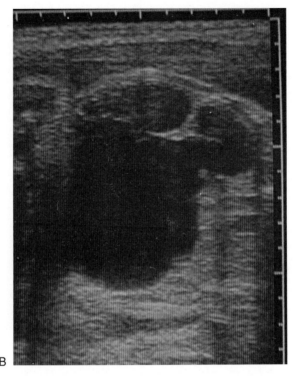

B

FIG. 12-22. *(Continued.)* **B:** Monitored later in gestation, the obstructed kidney continues to grow as illustrated here. Polyhydramnios and preterm labor are common complications of such a large abdominal mass. (*Source:* Reprinted from Seeds JW, Azizkhan RG. *Congenital Malformations: Antenatal Diagnosis, Perinatal Management, and Counseling.* Aspen Publishers, Inc. © 1990; p. 341.)

Urethral atresia results in obstruction from the earliest point in development. As early as 15 weeks, a large bladder with ascites is seen (Fig. 12-24). Later, the ascites resolves as the bladder continues to grow. The bladder remains symmetrical and discretely outlined. Oligohydramnios evolves and the kidneys appear initially small and echodense (Fig. 12-25), but later develop an enlarged, cystic pattern. Pulmonary hypoplasia is a virtual certainty. Attempts to divert urine and bypass the obstruction as early as 17 weeks have not prevented this outcome despite technical success.

Urethral Valves

Posterior urethral valves are essentially only a flimsy flap of tissue forming a valve within the urethra blocking the passage of urine. The results are catastrophic, although somewhat variable. Both the competence of the valves as ob-

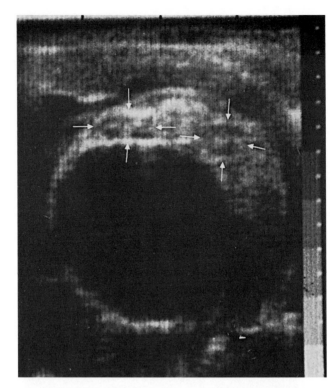

FIG. 12-23. If a weak area of the urinary tract above the obstruction expands to accept the urine, a large eccentric anechoic mass is produced as illustrated here. The *arrows* indicate the kidneys. This patient did present with polyhydramnios and preterm labor from this retroperitoneal urinoma. (*Source:* Reprinted from Seeds JW, Azizkhan RG. *Congenital Malformations: Antenatal Diagnosis, Perinatal Management, and Counseling.* Aspen Publishers, Inc. © 1990; p. 343.)

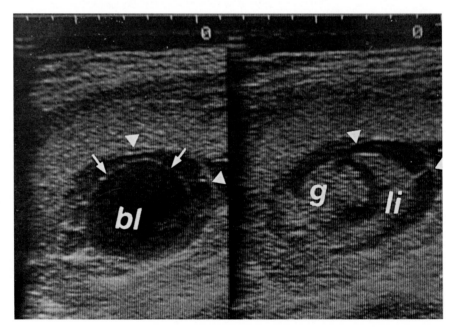

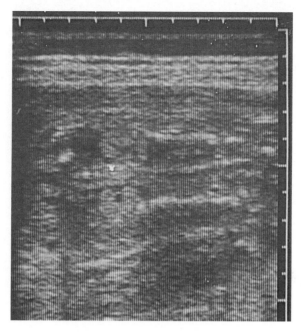

FIG. 12-25. In the case of very early obstruction such as urethral atresia, the kidneys appear echodense as shown here. Both kidneys are seen to be echodense on either side of the spine in this coronal view.

struction, and the time in gestation when the obstruction is accomplished may vary, resulting in variability of prognosis. Although up to 60% of these infants develop pulmonary hypoplasia and 80% show some degree of renal failure, the outcome is not so sure as with atresia, and several successes have been recorded with antenatal diversion drainage.

The sonographic appearance is that of a large bladder (Fig. 12-26), and bilateral moderate-to-severe hydronephrosis (Fig. 12-27) with caliectasis. Severe oligohydramnios is common but not absolute, since the degree and timing of the obstruction is variable.

Prune Belly Syndrome

The prune belly syndrome is often used to describe the appearance of a neonate born with urethral obstruction, megacystis, and, after drainage, the appearance of a prune belly. There is, however, a syndrome that includes megacystis, severe hy-

---

FIG. 12-24. Urethral atresia blocks the egress of urine from the beginning of urine production around 11 weeks. The result is a large bladder *(small arrows)* often within ascites *(triangles)*. In the image on the right, the gut *(g)* and the liver *(li)* may be seen. *bl,* bladder.

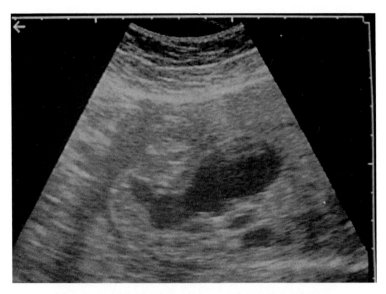

FIG. 12-26. The bladder, in the case of urethral valves, expands and fills the abdomen. This sagittal view shows the abdominal bladder to the right, the pelvic bladder to the left, extending into the posterior urethra ending in a point. The posterior urethra may be seen only in a sagittal scan.

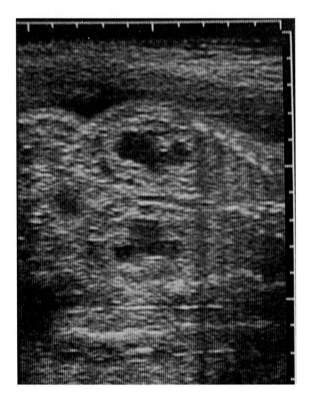

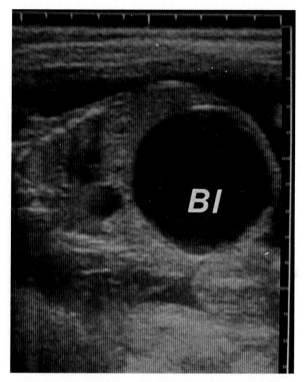

FIG. 12-28. This very large bladder *(Bl)* is found with normal-to-increased amniotic fluid. This apparent contradiction is characteristic of the prune belly syndrome, characterized by overflow voiding from a dysfunctional urinary tract. Severe hydronephrosis, hydroureter, and megacystis, associated with normal-to-increased amniotic fluid typifies the syndrome.

droureter and hydronephrosis (Fig. 12-28), agenesis of the rectus muscles, and undescended testicles without necessarily urethral obstruction. This syndrome is called the true *prune belly syndrome* and results from functional ureteral and bladder defects that produce the sonographic equivalent of obstruction, but oligohydramnios is not part of the condition. In fact, polyhydramnios is common.

The contradiction of a severely obstructed urinary tract sonographically with normal or often increased amniotic fluid volume is most likely prune belly syndrome. These babies typically do not develop pulmonary hypoplasia, and survival is expected.

FIG. 12-27. The kidneys here associated with urethral valves appear hydronephrotic. This coronal view shows both kidneys with hydronephrosis (dark, or anechoic areas) on either side of the midline.

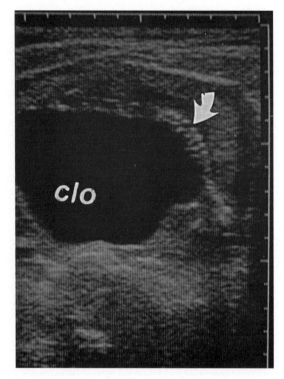

FIG. 12-29. Irregularity of outline characterizes the persistent cloaca *(clo)*. The functional equivalent of urethral atresia, renal dysplasia, and pulmonary hypoplasia are expected. (*Source:* Reprinted from Seeds JW, Azizkhan RG. *Congenital Malformations: Antenatal Diagnosis, Perinatal Management, and Counseling.* Aspen Publishers, Inc. © 1990; p. 355.)

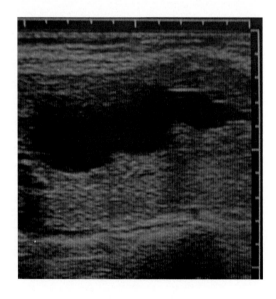

Cloacal Plate Malformation

Persistence of the embryonic cloaca that includes urinary tract and hindgut is often associated with obstruction and produces a large anechoic mass of the abdomen and anhydramnios (Fig. 12-29). Sonographically, this condition differs from simple urethral obstruction in that the anechoic mass is not symmetrical but instead irregular in outline (Fig. 12-30), since it is a combination of more than one organ system. The irregularity of outline is characteristic.

Pulmonary hypoplasia, renal dysplasia, and neonatal death are expected with cloacal plate syndrome, and antenatal diversion is not expected to benefit these infants.

MANAGEMENT OF THE URINARY TRACT MALFORMATION

Critical management issues include accurate diagnosis, assessment of fetal karyotype, gestational age at diagnosis, and prognosis or natural history of the condition in question.

In the case of bilateral renal agenesis or dysplasia, fetal or neonatal death are the result of pulmonary hypoplasia, and no alteration in perinatal management will change this outcome. Early attempts to divert fetal urine and provide for more normal development in the case of urethral atresia were technical successes but clinical failures, as the babies died regardless. On the other hand, in the case of unilateral disease including dysplasia or obstruction, with a normally functioning contralateral kidney, no alteration in management is likely to benefit the infant because the prognosis is so good.

The two urinary conditions that might benefit from antenatal intervention are posterior urethral valves and unilateral ureteropelvic junction obstruction resulting in a large eccentric abdominal mass causing polyhydramnios and preterm labor.

Multiple examples of apparent benefit from vesicoamniotic diversion in the case of posterior urethral valves have been reported. The most common method involves placement via percutaneous needles of a straight or a double pigtail catheter to drain urine from the bladder into the amniotic cavity. A similar technique may be used to drain the kidney or urinoma causing bowel displacement and polyhydramnios into the amniotic cavity. Alternatively, open laparotomy and hysterotomy followed by surgical fetal vesicostomy have been performed and reported, but the outcome is not clearly superior, and the trauma to the maternal uterus is substantial.

Fetal interventions cannot be undertaken without careful consideration and

FIG. 12-30. This is another example of a cloacal plate malformation, with multiple systems comprising the anechoic abdominal mass associated with anhydramnios. The irregularity of outline is apparent here. (*Source:* Reprinted from Seeds JW, Azizkhan RG. *Congenital Malformations: Antenatal Diagnosis, Perinatal Management, and Counseling.* Aspen Publishers, Inc. © 1990; p. 354.)

discussion of alternatives that include expectant management and early delivery. The experience of the clinical team is also important in such discussions.

In the case of bladder obstruction, various methods for assessment of renal function have been proposed, but none offer absolute diagnostic value. The osmolarity of the fetal urine has been proposed as a measure of fetal renal damage, with isosmotic urine suggesting renal damage and poor prognosis regardless of treatment. However, in the case of a very early gestational age, isosmotic fetal urine is the norm, so gestational age is important in this assessment. Furthermore, urine from a long-obstructed system may not represent current or potentially recoverable function if relief of the obstruction is provided. Therefore, fetal urine electrolyte or osmolarity values may or may not indicate the potential function of fetal kidneys.

Visual assessment of renal parenchyma is of some value. If the kidneys are small and echodense in early gestation, permanent renal damage is likely and benefit from antenatal or perinatal intervention is unlikely. Later in pregnancy, kidneys damaged by early obstructive uropathy show multiple, variable size parenchymal cysts.

A fetal karyotype is generally recommended in the case of any sonographic dysmorphology, and the urinary tract is no exception. Cells found in fetal urine are a good basis for karyotype. Drainage of the dilated bladder may serve two purposes. Not only to provide for a karyotype, but as a primitive test of function by an assessment of the rate of refilling.

Parents may choose only one of three options that include antenatal intervention, delivery, or expectant management. The choice is best based on an accurate diagnosis, a clear and accurate prognosis given no treatment, and the gestational age at the time of the decision. Careful counseling by a team of providers including genetic counselor, perinatologist, neonatologist, and pediatric surgeon is strongly recommended prior to any antenatal therapeutic interventions.

FURTHER READING

Arger P, Coleman B, Mintz M, Snyder H, Camardese T, Arenson R, Gabbe S, Aquino L. Routine fetal genitourinary tract screening. *Radiology* 1985;156:485–9.

Carpenter MW, Curci MR, Dibbins AW, Haddow JE. Perinatal management of ventral wall defects. *Obstet Gynecol* 1984;64:646.

Glick PL, Harrison MR, Golbus MS, *et al.* Management of the fetus with congenital hydronephrosis II. Prognostic criteria and selection for treatment. *J Ped Surg* 1985;20:376–87.

Hobbins J, Romero R, Grannum P, Berkowitz R, Cullen M, Mahoney M. Antenatal diagnosis of renal anomalies with ultrasound. *Am J Obstet Gynecol* 1984;148:868–77.

Kirk EP, Wah RM. Obstetric management of the fetus with omphalocele or gastroschisis: a review and report of one hundred twelve cases. *Am J Obstet Gynecol* 1983;146:512.

Manning FA, Harman CR, Lange IR, *et al.* Antepartum chronic fetal vesicoamniotic shunts for obstructive uropathy: a report of two cases. *Am J Obstet Gynecol* 1983;145:819–22.

Schaffer RM, Barone C, Friedman AP. The ultrasonographic spectrum of fetal omphalocele. *J Ultrasound Med* 1983;2:219.

Seeds JW, Cefalo RC, Herbert WNP, Bowes WA. Hydramnios and maternal renal failure: relief with fetal therapy. *Obstet Gynecol* 1984;64:26S.

13

Prenatal Diagnosis of Fetal Skeletal Malformations

There are more than 135 distinct congenital long bone dysplasias. They are rare, with the aggregate incidence only about 1–3 per thousand live births. The majority result in only mild or moderate shortening of limbs, while others are severe and debilitating or even lethal. Some attention to examination of long bones should be included in every obstetrical ultrasound examination. Measurement of femur length (Fig. 13-1) is an accepted part of fetal biometry for both dating and estimating fetal weight, and it is an accepted screening dimension for a patient not known to be at increased risk for short limb dysplasias. For any patient known to be at increased risk, imaging, if not measurement, of all long bones is recommended.

Long bone dysplasias commonly cause limbs to be shorter than expected, but many also result in altered bone density, strength, and shape. Although ultrasound cannot reliably assess density, length and shape are easily evaluated. Curvature or sharp angulation that indicates fracture are clues to the type of dysplasia in question (Fig. 13-2). Many long bone dysplasias are associated with other predictable skeletal deformities such as deformities of the cranium or chest. A cloverleaf skull (Fig. 13-3), an easily deformed cranium (Fig. 13-4), or a virtually transparent cranium sonographically may lead to a specific diagnosis. Lethality is typically the result of thoracic dystrophy related to short ribs that result in pulmonary hypoplasia (Fig. 13-5). Therefore, the chest assessment may be helpful in categorizing the condition.

Milder forms of certain dysplasias may not be sufficiently apparent in early pregnancy to allow diagnosis prior to the midpoint of gestation, while others are detectable with reasonable confidence.

A sensitive and accurate approach to the screening and diagnosis of short limb dysplasias begins with a review of the normal anatomy, an examination of the limits of normal, and a discussion of certain unique characteristics of selected conditions.

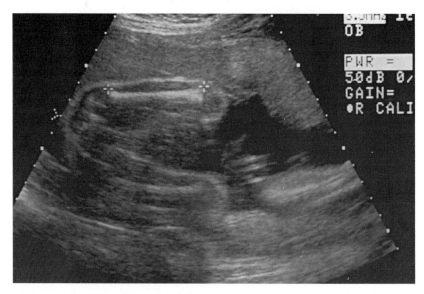

FIG. 13-1. After careful attention to full capture of the entire length of the fetal femur, the bone is measured from blunt endpoint to blunt endpoint, parallel to the shaft.

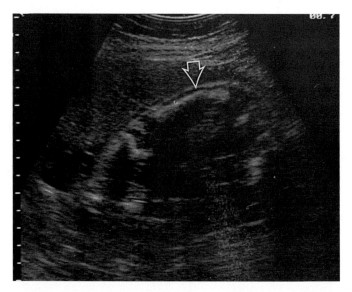

FIG. 13-2. This femur demonstrates an abrupt angulation *(arrow)* characteristic of a severe form of osteogenesis imperfecta. (*Source:* Reprinted from Seeds JW, Azizkhan RG. *Congenital Malformations: Antenatal Diagnosis, Perinatal Management, and Counseling.* Aspen Publishers, Inc. © 1990; p. 164.)

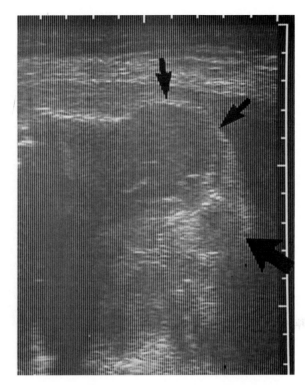

FIG. 13-3. The characteristic bulging and deformity of the cloverleaf skull (*large arrow* indicates orbit, *smaller arrows* denote bulging of skull behind orbits) is a clue to the specific diagnosis. This fetus was found to have achondrogenesis. (*Source:* Reprinted from Seeds JW, Azizkhan RG. *Congenital Malformations: Antenatal Diagnosis, Perinatal Management, and Counseling.* Aspen Publishers, Inc. © 1990; p. 160.)

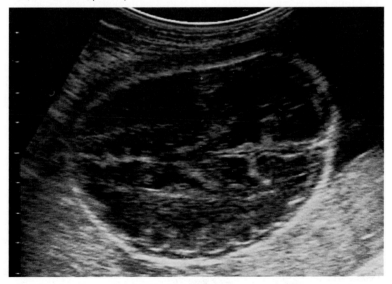

FIG. 13-4. The suspicious transparency and easy deformability of this cranium suggests bone dysplasia. These characteristics are typical for osteogenesis imperfecta.

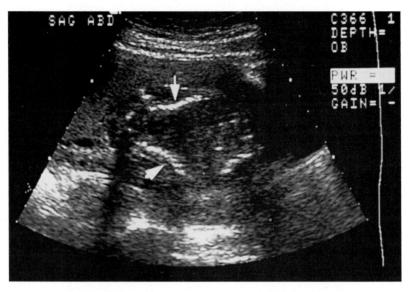

FIG. 13-5. The small chest that is associated with many lethal short limb dysplasias causes a narrowing of the chest above the abdomen *(arrows)*, a crowding of the heart, and compression of the lungs.

NORMAL ANATOMY

All fetal long bones may be seen with realtime ultrasound and measured from 12 weeks to term. The femur is perhaps the easiest to capture and measure due to its more limited range of motion and is, therefore, the long bone most often measured. However, all fetal long bones demonstrate a close and reproducible relationship to gestational age. Growth of the femur and the other long bones has been reported to be nearly linear through early pregnancy with a slowly diminishing slope in later stages. Furthermore, there is a nearly linear relationship between all the long bones and the biparietal diameter (BPD).

Through the critical diagnostic period of 14–22 weeks, all the long bones may be compared with a screening chart (Table 13-1).

The imaging of the femur may start from the transverse trunk or longitudinal spinal scanplanes. From the transverse trunk, slide the transducer caudal, and the femur will be crossed transversely as it is typically flexed on the hip (Fig. 13-6). Once found transversely, the transducer is rotated until the entire length is seen (Fig. 13-7A,B). From the longitudinal spinal plane, the transducer is moved longitudinally caudally to the coccyx, then rotated ventrally about a quarter turn until some part of the femur is seen, then developed. Special care is necessary to insure that the entire length of the bone is captured. Unclear endpoints without good landmarks suggest the possibility that the scanplane does not include the entire bone and that any measurement, therefore, would underestimate the true

TABLE 13–1. *Long bone dimensions in early gestation (mm)*

Gestational age	± 4.3 mm (95% CI)			
	Femur	Humerus	Tibia/Fibula	Radius/Ulna
14	14	15	12	12
16	20	20	16	17
18	26	25	22	21
20	32	31	27	26
22	38	36	32	30

FL = −29.49 ± 3.09 (GA)
GA = FL + 29.49/3.09
CI, confidence level; FL, femur length; GA, gestational age.

bone length. The acoustical shadowing characteristic of the diaphyseal shaft can help in truly defining the endpoints for measurement.

The visible femur extends from metaphyseal plate to metaphyseal plate. The sonographic image does not include the cartilaginous epiphyseal areas and therefore underestimates the palpable length of the bone by 8–17%, depending on gestational age. This undermeasurement is not clinically relevant for diagnosis, since any individual dimension is empirically compared with a normal reference database determined in a comparable fashion. It is important not to include in

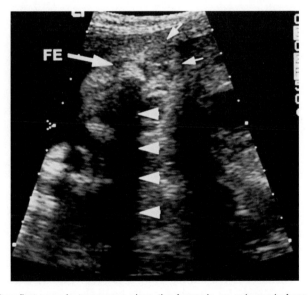

FIG. 13-6. Often first seen in transverse view, the femur is an echogenic focus *(large arrow)* within the thigh *(small arrows)*. The femur casts a dense acoustic shadow *(arrowheads).*

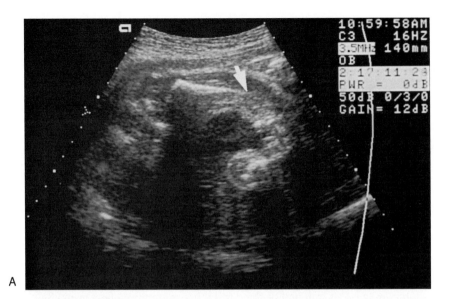

A

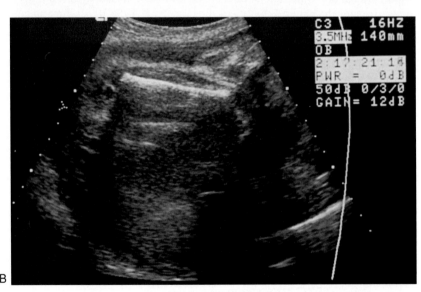

B

FIG. 13-7. A: Rotation of the transducer will show progressively greater length of the femur, but in this case the image is incomplete as one terminus ends without a distinct blunt landmark *(arrow)*. Further adjustment of the scanplane is necessary to capture the full length of the bone. **B:** Full capture of the femur is indicated by symmetrical blunt landmarks with acoustic shadows.

your measurement the occasional linear echo extension of the near surface that represents a specular echo from the proximal surface of the epiphysis.

Measurement is parallel to the shaft of the bone shaft from metaphyseal plate to metaphyseal plate. Shadows should be dense and sharply defined. Endpoints should be clear and blunt. It is recommended that the bone be as parallel to the transducer surface as possible to avoid any error due to differential sound speed through tissues.

Images of the fetal femur and humerus (Fig. 13-8A,B) appear similar, and their length is similar in early gestation. The femur is less mobile and therefore easier to capture, but the growth relationships are equally precise. The tibia and fibula, and the radius and ulna, also appear similar (Fig. 13-9A,B), but imaging of these

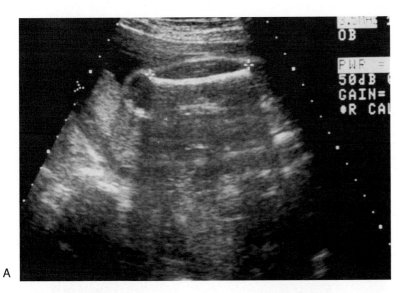

A

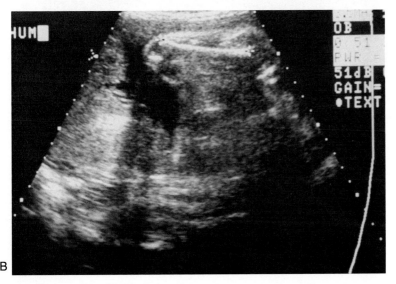

B

FIG. 13-8. A: The normal femur in full image with acoustic shadows. **B:** The full humerus from the same fetus as in Fig. 13-8A. Note the similarity of shape and size in early gestation.

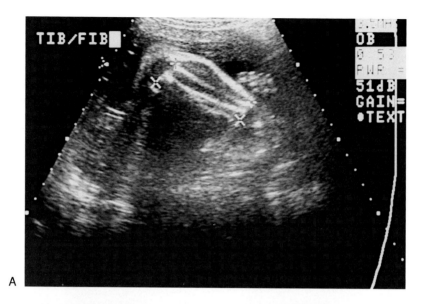

A

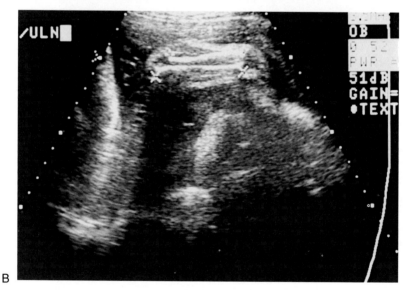

B

FIG. 13-9. A: The tibia and fibula may be seen together if the scanplane is manipulated to place them in a coplanar relationship. **B:** The radius and ulna may also be seen together in a coplanar scan.

requires more time and effort and is typically reserved for those cases known to be at risk, or in those in which other findings suggest pathology.

GROWTH RELATIONSHIPS

There are a variety of different long bone/gestational age reference charts available, and no two are identical. All charts appeared correct to the reporting author. It is for the individual practitioner to validate a particular chart for himself with his or her own sonographic and clinical experience. The simplest validation would include the recording of fetal biometric parameters for each fetus for a period of 3–6 months, and a review of the correlation of estimated gestational ages between parameters and between the average for a fetus and the clinical age of the fetus. A consistent or average negative or positive discrepancy would alert the clinician to the possibility that either the technique or the chart used may be in error.

Most investigators have found the relationship early in gestation to be linear but charts (Table 13-1) are easier to use. During the 14–22-week interval, the femur is expected to grow about 3 mm per week. The expected limits of normal are about plus or minus a week and a half, or 4.3 mm. However, the diagnosis of a short limb dysplasia is more complex than simply measuring a femur to be 4.4 mm short for gestational age. Accuracy of the clinical gestational age, compatibility with other fetal dimensions, shape of long bones, shape of cranium, size and appearance of the chest, and familial stature characteristics must be taken into account. Furthermore, the very nature of a 95% confidence interval implies that one out of twenty individuals lies outside these limits.

The relationship between fetal long bones and BPD is linear throughout gestation. This allows the observer to index a given measurement to the fetus itself and not to a clinical gestational age that might be in error.

$$BPD = -9.79 + .864(FL) \ (\pm 5.3 \ 95\% \ CI)$$

$$BPD = -4.94 + .73 \ (Hu) \ (\pm 5.7 \ 95\% \ CI)$$

Another internal control is femur-to-foot length ratio. Most investigators have found that the fetal femur is only slightly longer on average than the fetal foot (Fig. 13-10) in early gestation and shorter in the third trimester giving the observer another convenient internal standard. The femur length in the third trimester should not be less than 85% of the foot length in the normal case. In the case of most serious dwarf conditions, this comparison demonstrates significant deviation from this expected relationship.

If, during the screening examination, the femur appears to lag behind the clinical gestational age and/or other fetal dimension, a short limb dysplasia may be suspected. Consideration of familial stature is important, but other comparisons are useful. Measure the foot length. Subtract 10% from the foot length in early gestation, and 15% in the third trimester. If the femur length exceeds 90% of the

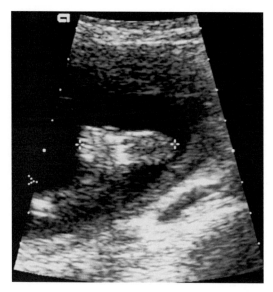

FIG. 13-10. Follow the leg to the foot, rotate the scanplane to capture the full plantar surface of the foot, and measure the full length of the foot from heel to toe, as illustrated here, to provide a dimension for internal comparison to femur length. With some practice this image is not difficult.

foot length in early gestation, and 85% in the third trimester, the apparent lag is probably familial short stature, not a long bone dysplasia. Compare the measured femur length to the expected average, and, typically, the difference is less than 10 mm, reassuring the patient. Furthermore, assess the shape of the long bones and look at the chest. Lethal long bone dysplasias typically cause thoracodystrophy. If the heart-to-chest relationships appear normal, then most of these severe conditions are excluded (Fig. 13-11A,B,C).

An adequate evaluation of the fetus suspected of a short limb dysplasia, then, would include a variety of elements (Table 13-2).

TABLE 13–2. *Elements of the sonographic examination of a fetus at risk for long bone dysplasia*

Long bone length
Long bone shape
Cranial shape and dimensions
Foot length
Chest evaluation to include circumference, relationship of four
  chamber heart circumference to chest circumference
Family stature

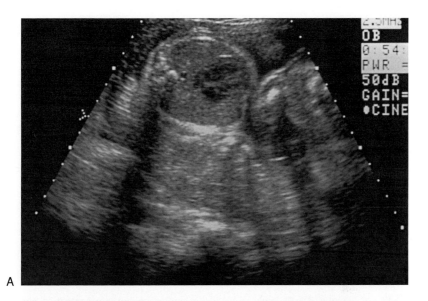

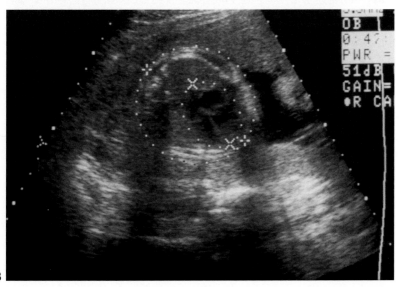

FIG. 13-11. A: The normal four-chamber view allows the examiner to subjectively judge that the cardiac area is about one third of the chest area, and at least no greater than one half. Also note that the cardiac long axis is inclined to the midline at 45 degrees and that the midline crosses the left atrium and exits the right ventricle. **B:** Most equipment allows the examiner to precisely measure these relationships if subjective assessment suggests a question.

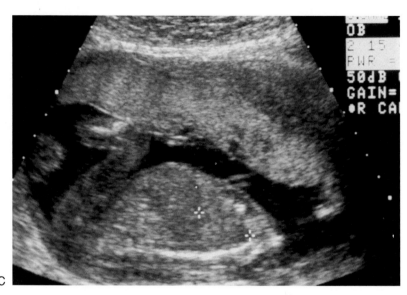

FIG. 13-11. *(Continued)* **C:** Recently, investigators have found that lung length from diaphragm to apex *(cursors)* bears a strong relationship to lung development and may become useful in assessing the possibility of hypoplasia.

SHORT LIMB DYSPLASIAS

Prenatal diagnosis of short limb dysplasia allows for planned delivery and parental preparation, and accurate diagnosis allows for accurate family planning counseling. The early diagnosis of severe, disabling, or lethal dysplasias may allow the parents to consider other options. The official nomenclature for long bone dysplasias is cumbersome and not all that necessary for an adequate clinical understanding of these conditions (Table 13-3).

The indication for prenatal diagnosis is based on a clinical assessment of the risk of affectation (Table 13-4). Short limb dysplasias may be lethal or not (Table

TABLE 13–3. *Nomenclature of long bone dysplasias*

Acromelia	Shortening of distal segments
Mesomelia	Shortening of middle segments
Micromelia	Shortened extremities
Rhizomelia	Shortening of proximal segments
Phocomelia	Absent or short middle segments
Sirenomelia	Fusion of the legs
Clinodactyly	Overlapping digits

TABLE 13–4. *Indications for prenatal diagnosis of short limb dysplasias*

Previously affected child
Affected parent
Polyhydramnios: Many forms of congenital dwarfism associated with polyhydramnios including:
    camptomelic dysplasia
    thanatophoric dysplasia
    achondroplasia
    asphyxiating thoracodystrophy
    hypophosphatasia
    achondrogenesis
Short limbs noted at ultrasound done for other purposes.

TABLE 13–5. *Lethal short limb dwarf conditions*

Thanatophoric dysplasia
Achondrogenesis
Osteogenesis imperfecta type II
Hypophosphatasia
Chondrodysplasia punctata
Camptomelic dysplasia

13-5). Lethal dwarf conditions as mentioned above, most often produce a compressed, narrow thorax that results in pulmonary hypoplasia.

In the case of a fetus suspected of a short limb condition, it may be difficult to distinguish certain specific conditions from other, similar dysplasias. The exact diagnosis may or may not be possible until the infant is born. In the vast majority of cases, however, the clinician will be able to answer the patient's most pressing questions: Is the baby going to look abnormal? Is the baby likely to live? With or without disabilities?

DIAGNOSTIC TECHNIQUES

Ultrasound

The average bone length for a given gestational age ± 2 SD includes about 95% of the population. Even though the identification of a fetus with a femur at or just outside these limits raises the suspicion of a dwarf condition, be careful. Familial short stature will occasionally produce such an outlier, while most serious dwarf conditions are far below the expected dimensional limits, not close to them.

Certain conditions characteristically show bowing (Fig. 13-12), others may show antenatal fractures (Table 13-6). Most lethal conditions show serious narrowing of the chest cavity (Fig. 13-13), and are therefore associated with pulmonary hypoplasia (Table 13-7). Hypomineralization of the bones characterizes a relative few, but severe, conditions (Table 13-8).

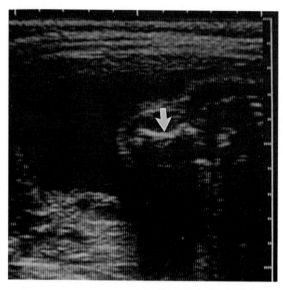

FIG. 13-12. The bowing as well as the shortening of this femur *(arrow)* of a fetus with camptomelic dysplasia is characteristic. (*Source:* Reprinted from Seeds JW, Azizkhan RG. *Congenital Malformations: Antenatal Diagnosis, Perinatal Management, and Counseling.* Aspen Publishers, Inc. © 1990; p. 162.)

In the case of osteogenesis imperfecta (OI), bone density may not appear altered with ultrasound, but in the case of the fetus affected by hypophosphatasia or achondrogenesis, the skeleton is essentially invisible to ultrasound (Fig. 13-14). The striking image of a fetal spine without visible bony elements should alert the examiner to this possibility. The severe forms of OI are characterized by *in utero* fractures that produce abrupt angulation of the long bone (Fig. 13-15A,B).

Radiography may be useful at or after 19 weeks and can be helpful in assessing fetal bone density and shape. In many cases, radiographic confirmation is unnecessary, however, since distinct and clear characteristics of a particular diagnosis are often available with ultrasound.

TABLE 13–6. *Conditions associated with either fractures or bowing of long bones*

Achondrogenesis
Camptomelic dysplasia
Hypophosphatasia
Osteogenesis imperfecta (OI) type II, III
Thanatophoric dysplasia

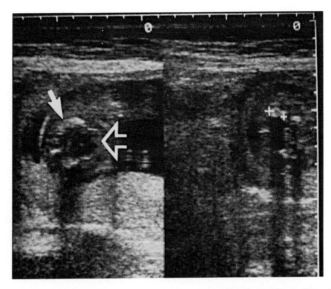

FIG. 13-13. The severe disproportion of heart *(open arrow)* to chest *(arrow)* on the left, combined with the severe shortening of the femur on the right (11 mm at 20 weeks) are characteristic of severe short limb dysplasias associated with thoracodystrophy. (*Source:* Reprinted from Seeds JW, Azizkhan RG. *Congenital Malformations: Antenatal Diagnosis, Perinatal Management, and Counseling.* Aspen Publishers, Inc. © 1990; p. 161.)

Amniography was used historically to assess fetal surface soft tissue anatomy by injecting dye into the amniotic fluid prior to radiographic study. The technique has been replaced by ultrasound.

Risk to the pregnancy from diagnostic testing should always be considered. Although no known methodologic danger is associated with ultrasound, an indirect danger arises from errors in diagnosis. Minimal risk of carcinogenesis from radiography alone or with amniography is known.

Diagnostic error may arise if minor discrepancies are used as the basis for a major diagnosis without a careful assessment of familial stature or the other complementary diagnostic observations. A diagnosis may not be made if the condition is not manifest early in pregnancy, as is the case with many milder conditions such as heterozygous achondroplasia or OI types I and IV.

TABLE 13–7. *Conditions associated with thoracodystrophy*

Thanatophoric dysplasia
Achondrogenesis
Hypophosphatasia
Camptomelic dysplasia
Asphyxiating thoracodystrophy

TABLE 13–8. *Conditions associated with hypomineralization*

Osteogenesis imperfecta
Hypophosphatasia
Achondrogenesis

The sonographer, therefore, must look at more than the bone length. A careful evaluation of those features included in Table 13-9 is recommended in the case of any fetus considered to be at risk. Among reports of successful antenatal diagnoses of severe forms of long bone dysplasia, over 70% had one of four specific diagnoses:

> thanatophoric dwarf
> osteogenesis imperfecta
> achondrogenesis
> achondroplasia

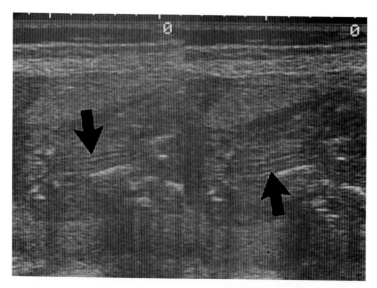

FIG. 13-14. These longitudinal views of the spine of a fetus with achondrogenesis demonstrate the transparency of the fetal skeleton in this hypomineralization condition. (*Source:* Reprinted from Seeds JW, Azizkhan RG. *Congenital Malformations: Antenatal Diagnosis, Perinatal Management, and Counseling.* Aspen Publishers, Inc. © 1990; p. 160.)

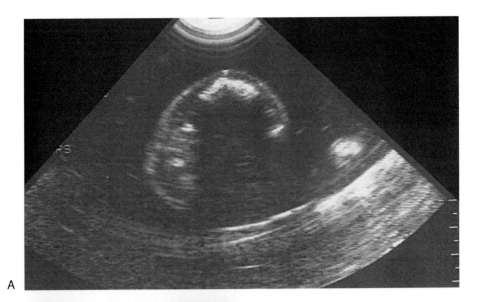

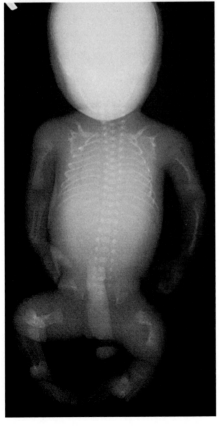

FIG. 13-15. A: The sharp angulation of this femur is characteristic of one of the severe forms of osteogenesis imperfecta. **B:** The radiograph of a fetus with a severe form of osteogenesis imperfecta shows multiple fractures and severe attenuation of the growth of the long bones.

TABLE 13–9. *Elements of evaluation of short limb dysplasia*

Degree of shortening
Distribution of shortening
Presence of fractures
Degree of echogenicity
Shape and echogenicity of calvarium
Shape and size of thorax
Presence of polydactyly

SPECIFIC SELECTED CONDITIONS

Thanatophoric Dysplasia

This is the most common form of lethal dwarfism. The sonographer will find marked shortening of bowed long bones and a small chest. The condition is lethal because of pulmonary hypoplasia, and it is considered nongenetic with a low recurrence risk. A small minority have cloverleaf skull and these cases may demonstrate autosomal recessive pattern.

Achondrogenesis

This is the second most common severe lethal short limb dysplasia. It is marked with short long bones, the majority of which have poor ossification of the vertebrae but good ossification of the calvarium, which distinguishes it from hypophosphatasia in which the calvarium is as poorly mineralized as the rest of the spinal column. Polyhydramnios is common. A 25% risk of recurrence indicates autosomal recessive inheritance.

Asphyxiating Thoracodystrophy

Markedly short long bones, an extremely small funnel-shaped chest, and polyhydramnios mark this form of long bone dysplasia characterized by neonatal death due to pulmonary hypoplasia.

Camptomelic Dysplasia

This severe form shows markedly short, bowed, long bones, with the lower limbs more severely affected, and polyhydramnios is common. This condition is variably survivable.

Chondroectodermal Dysplasia

This condition shows short limbs and polydactyly, indicating the value of examination of the fetal hands in the diagnosis of limb dysplasia. This form shows a low recurrence risk.

Diastrophic Dwarfism

This is a nonlethal condition with short limbs, spinal deformities, and normal intelligence. This form of dwarfism is inherited in an autosomal recessive pattern.

Osteogenesis Imperfecta

OI comes in at least four forms with significantly differing characteristics:

Type I: milder, survivable, autosomal dominant
Type II: severe, lethal, marked shortening, fractures, autosomal recessive
Type III: severe, marked shortening, fractures, survivable for variable time, autosomal recessive
Type IV: milder, survivable, autosomal dominant with unlikely diagnosis early.

The identification of a sharply angulated long bone indicates a fracture and indicates osteogensis imperfecta. *In utero* fractures are not seen with other long bone dysplasias.

Achondroplasia

The most common type of unexpected congenital dwarfism occurs in families with normal parents as a result of acute mutation. It is most often mild, and prenatal diagnosis by ultrasound at 22 weeks is possible. But normal or near-normal bone lengths earlier than 22 weeks prevent conclusive detection. Growth typically crosses percentiles, so serial observation is suggested. Achondroplasia is autosomal dominant, so there is a 50% risk of affectation in the children of an affected parent, but only a slightly higher risk of recurrence to normal parents based on acute mutation.

Robert's Syndrome

When renal dysplasia, tetraphocomelia, oligohydramnios, and no bladder filling are combined, Robert's syndrome may be suspected. This is lethal due to pulmonary hypoplasia and carries a 25% recurrence.

Hypophosphatasia

Nonmineralization of entire skeleton with nonvisualization on ultrasound as well as radiographs suggests hypophosphatasia. Markedly short limbs are combined with a small chest, and the condition is lethal.

SUMMARY

Visualization and measurement of the femurs should be a part of every obstetrical ultrasound examination. Imaging if not measurement of all long bones should be considered if a pregnancy is known to be at increased risk of a short limb dysplasia. Diagnosis of a short limb condition on the basis of a measurement alone that is below but near the lower limits of normal should be suspect. Any suspicion should lead to an assessment of the cranium, the chest, amniotic fluid, digits, and serial assessment. The identification of diminished density, curvature, angulation or fracture, thoracodystrophy, or cranial deformity, strongly supports the diagnosis of a significant short limb dysplasia.

FURTHER READING

Aylsworth AS, Seeds JW, Guildford WB, *et al.* Prenatal diagnosis of a severe deforming type of osteogensis imperfecta. *Am J Med Gen* 1984;19:707.

Golbus MS, Hall BD, Filly RA, Poskanzer LB. Prenatal diagnosis of achondrogenesis. *J Pediatr* 1977;91: 464.

Hobbins JC, Bracken MB, Mahoney MJ. Diagnosis of fetal skeletal dysplasias with ultrasound. *Am J Obstet Gynecol* 1982;142:306.

Kaitila I, Ammala P, Karjalainen O, *et al.* Early prenatal detection of diastrophic dysplasia. *Prenatal Diagnosis* 1983;3:237.

Kurtz AB, Wapner RJ. Ultrasonographic diagnosis of second trimester skeletal dysplasias: a prospective analysis in a high risk populatiion. *J Ultrasound Med* 1983;2:99.

Mahoney BS, Filly RA. High resolution sonographic assessment of the fetal extremities. *J Ultrasound Med* 1984;3:489.

Nimrod C, Davies D, Iwanicki S, *et al* Ultrasound prediction of pulmonary hypoplasia. *Obstet Gynecol* 1986;68:495.

Seeds JW, Cefalo RC. Relationship of fetal limb lengths to both biparietal diameter and gestational age. *Obstet Gynecol* 1982;60:680.

Shaff MI, Fleischer AC, Battino R, *et al.* Antenatal sonographic diagnosis of thanatophoric dysplasia. *J Clin Ultrasound* 1980;8:363.

Skiptunas SM, Weiner S. Early prenatal diagnosis of asphyxiating thoracic dystrophy Jeune's syndrome. *J Ultrasound Med* 1987;6:41.

Wong WS, Filly RA. Polyhydramnios associated with fetal limb abnormalities. *AJF* 1983;140:1001.

14

Ectopic Pregnancy and Early Pregnancy Failure

Realtime ultrasound offers the opportunity to assess the status of the first-trimester pregnancy. Familiarity with early pregnancy anatomy and embryology will allow the practitioner to establish an accurate diagnosis in the vast majority of patients. In addition, correlation of ultrasound findings with the concentration of human chorionic gonadotropin (hCG) will frequently allow the early diagnosis of pregnancy failure or extrauterine implantation. This chapter will address the use of realtime ultrasound in the ambulatory setting for the evaluation of the first-trimester pregnancy.

EARLY PREGNANCY ANATOMY AND EMBRYOLOGY

The earliest change in uterine anatomy due to pregnancy is also the most subtle. The change from the proliferative to secretory phase endometrium secondary to the effects of progesterone results in an increased echogenicity of the endometrial echo. In early pregnancy, the decidualization of the endometrium resulting from stimulation by corpus luteal hormones results in a very echogenic endometrium. This change is subtle and, although characteristic, it is not diagnostic of early pregnancy.

During this period, the fertilized zygote traverses the fallopian tube and implants in the endometrium as a blastocyst. Following gastrulation of the zygote, the trilaminar embryonic disc develops on the dorsal surface of the yolk sac, and the amnion begins to delaminate from the dorsal surface of the disc. The surrounding trophoblastic epithelium encases all of the embryonic structures and eventually interfaces with the maternal circulation via the terminal trophoblastic villi.

The first definitive sign of pregnancy is the appearance of the gestational sac, which is made up of the embryonic disc, yolk sac, amnion, extra-coelomic fluid, and the surrounding trophoblastic membrane. The interface of fluid, trophoblastic tissue, and decidualized endometrium allows the sonographic detection of an early pregnancy as early as 2.5 weeks following conception.

The diagnosis of very small gestational sacs must be made with caution. Occasionally, a small decidual hematoma in the setting of an extrauterine pregnancy can mimic a small intrauterine gestational sac. The true gestational sac should exhibit the echogenic rim of the trophoblastic membrane. This finding can be subtle in extremely small gestational sacs (Fig. 14-1).

The normal gestational sac has been described in a variety of terms in an effort to characterize the presence of the trophoblastic membrane and decidual interface. The "double decidual sac sign" or "sac within a sac" are examples of this descriptive effort. Regardless of the terminology used, it is incumbent upon the sonographer/sonologist to verify and document the presence of the normal embryologic structures prior to unequivocally diagnosing an intrauterine anechoic area as a gestational sac.

Transabdominal and/or transvaginal scanning will allow assessment of the early pregnancy. The ability to approximate the early pregnancy with the transvaginal transducer results in improved resolution and a more definitive study.

The embryonic disc should be visualized in gestational sacs with a mean sac diameter in excess of 1.2 cm using the transvaginal approach. If transabdominal scanning is used, the embryonic pole should be seen with a mean sac diameter of 2.5 cm (Fig. 14-2). Once the embryonic length reaches 0.5 cm, embryonic cardiac flicker should be seen via transvaginal scanning. An embryonic length of 0.9

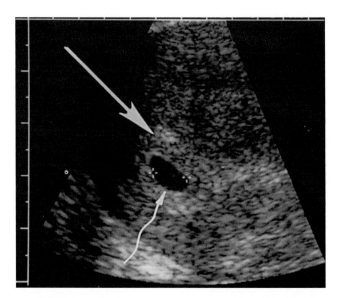

FIG. 14-1. The interface between the fluid within the early gestational sac and the surrounding endometrium allows the visualization of an early intrauterine pregnancy. Note the fluffy echogenicity of the decidualized endometrium *(straight arrow)* surrounding the echogenic chorionic echo *(curved arrow)* in this transvaginal image of a gestational sac of 6.5 mm.

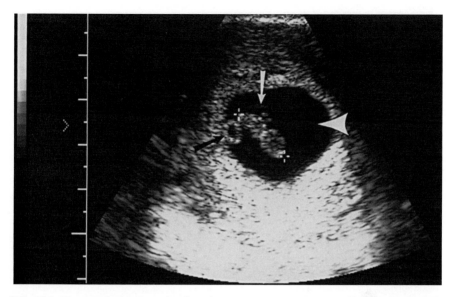

FIG. 14-2. Transvaginal image of a first-trimester pregnancy demonstrating the crown-rump length measurement *(+ calipers),* yolk sac *(black arrow),* amnion *(small white arrow),* and the extraembryonic coelomic space between the amnion and chorion *(large white arrowhead).*

cm should exhibit a visible embryonic cardiac flicker using transabdominal ultrasound techniques.

As the pregnancy advances, other embryonic structures will be apparent. The trophoblastic membrane will differentiate into a thin, relatively avascular membrane called the *chorion laeve.* The remainder of the surrounding membrane exhibits proliferation of trophoblastic villi and is designated the chorion frondosum. This structure will become the placenta and, eventually, become highly vascularized.

The embryonic disc enlarges and a cephalic pole, caudal pole, limb buds, and yolk sac may be easily discerned by 8 weeks (menstrual age). The amnion appears as a membrane surrounding the embryo, and the extraembryonic space between the amnion and chorion is readily visible (Fig. 14-3).

The sequential appearance of multiple embryologic landmarks has been thoroughly delineated. Many of these structures will be discussed in more detail in the section addressing early diagnosis of fetal anomalies.

Initially, normal fetal cardiac rate approximates the maternal rate. Merchiers noted a mean cardiac rate of 82 beats per minute (bpm) at 5 menstrual weeks but a rapid increase to mean rate of 156 bpm at 9 weeks. He also noted the ominous finding of declining fetal cardiac rate.

The presence of normal cardiac activity offers a very favorable prognosis for the pregnancy. Indeed, spontaneous abortion is uncommon following the appearance of normal fetal cardiac activity. A spontaneous loss rate of 8.8% fol-

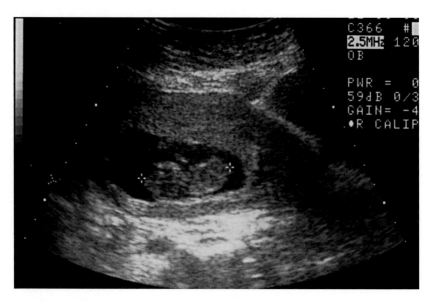

FIG. 14-3. A more advanced first-trimester image depicting an embryonic length of 41.4 mm *(calipers).*

lowing the detection of normal cardiac activity was reported in an analysis of 510 first-trimester patients with visible cardiac activity by Frates *et al.*

The measurement of the length of the embryo by establishing the crown-rump length allows determination of gestational age. The reliability of gestational age assignment was noted to be ±4.7 days (±1 SD) by Robinson *et al.*

DIAGNOSIS OF ABNORMAL PREGNANCY

In a normal pregnancy, the gestational sac should be visualized concomitantly with a concentration of hCG in maternal serum of 3000 mIU/ml [First International Reference Preparation (IRP) or "Third" World Health Organization (WHO) standard]. A discriminatory zone of 1800–2000 mIU/ml is effective unless a multifetal pregnancy is present. The higher value has been selected to allow a reliable discriminator even if a multifetal conception is present.

Failure to visualize a gestational sac with hCG concentrations above this critical concentration implies the presence of a pathologic pregnancy including the possibility of an abnormal intrauterine or extrauterine pregnancy.

As noted above, once the gestational sac has reached a mean sac diameter of 1.2 cm by transvaginal scanning or 2.5 cm by the transabdominal approach, the embryonic disc should be visible. When the embryonic disc measures 0.5 cm (vaginal scan) or 0.9 cm (abdominal scan) embryonic cardiac motion should be detectable.

TABLE 14–1. *Correlation of embryonic events visible by transvaginal ultrasound in normal uterine pregnancy*

hCG (mIU/ml 1st IRP)	Sac	Yolk sac	Flicker
<1,000	±	−	−
1,000–7,200	+	±	−
7,200–10,800	+	+	±
>10,800	+	+	+

Modified from Bree RL, Marn CS. Transvaginal sonography in the first trimester: embryology, anatomy, and hCG correlation. *Seminars in Ultrasound, CT, and MRI.* 1990;11:12–21.

Bree has attempted to establish the hCG concentration at which specific embryonic events should be seen. His data are summarized in Table 14-1.

Failure to visualize embryonic echoes in gestational sacs above the critical size allows the diagnosis of an anembryonic pregnancy or what was previously referred to as a *blighted ovum*. Likewise, the presence of an embryonic disc of sufficient size with no embryonic cardiac activity is compatible with the diagnosis of early embryonic demise.

The mean gestational sac diameter is calculated by averaging the three diameters of the sac. The relationship of the mean sac diameter to the crown-rump length has been evaluated for its prognostic potential. In a study of 539 pregnancies a mean sac diameter minus crown-rump length difference of <5 mm was noted to predict a poor prognosis with a spontaneous abortion frequency of 80%. When this difference was ≥8 mm only 49 of 461 pregnancies were lost.

An irregular or partially collapsed gestational sac is compatible with the diagnosis of an incomplete spontaneous abortion. These sacs may exhibit a variety of appearances depending upon the gestational age of the pregnancy, the amount of retained tissue, and the amount of bleeding that has occurred.

Gestational trophoblastic disease frequently presents as a hydatidiform mole. Whereas earlier sonographic descriptions of the "snowstorm" appearance of an advanced hydatidiform mole was an excellent descriptor of the image from static scanners, the usual diagnosis of hydatidiform mole using realtime equipment is usually characterized by numerous disorganized echoes depicting the multiple interfaces of the vesicular chorionic villi. In the first trimester, hydatidiform moles can appear as intrauterine gestational sacs with subtle abnormalities. These gestational sacs usually have abnormally thickened and/or disorganized placental echoes. Correlation with hCG concentration may be of benefit in the early diagnosis of the hydatidiform mole. It must be stressed that gestational trophoblastic disease may present a variety of appearances.

Retromembranous (subchorionic) hematomas are frequently encountered in the first trimester of pregnancy. Occasionally, these may be retroplacental in location. Large hematomatas and/or those that are retroplacental are associated

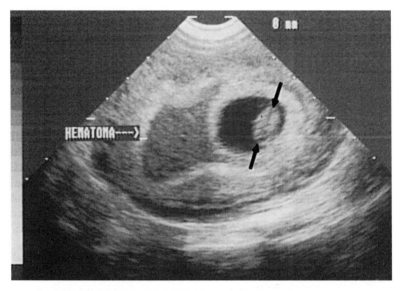

FIG. 14-4. A large intrauterine hematoma is noted juxtaposed to a first-trimester pregnancy. Note the homogeneous, ground-glass appearance of the hematoma. The chorion is very echogenic, and the fetal echo is clearly seen *(black arrows).*

with a poorer prognosis than those that are small and/or those that are subchorionic but do not involve the implantation site. Regardless of the size or location of the hematoma, an expectant management posture is justified as long as cardiac activity is present (Fig. 14-4).

EXTRAUTERINE PREGNANCY

The ability to diagnose extrauterine (ectopic) pregnancies in the preclinical phase has been a major advance in gynecology. Not only does this allow the opportunity to decrease morbidity and mortality, but also the entire concept of appropriate management has shifted to a more conservative approach and, in many cases, medical therapy. Correlation of sonographic findings with the concentration of hCG allows the diagnosis of abnormal pregnancy very early in the process in at-risk patients.

Human chorionic gonadotropin from the trophoblast increases rapidly during the first trimester. The use of two different reference preparations has resulted in some confusion regarding critical values. The First IRP and the WHO standard are similar. The Second International Reference Standard (Second IRS) results in values approximately one half of the other standard reference preparations. Therefore, a value of 3000 mIU/ml of the First IRP or WHO standard is equivalent to approximately 1500 mIU/ml of the second IRS. The values referred to in this chapter will refer to the First IRP.

The visualization of a normal gestational sac using transabdominal sonography should be possible with an hCG concentration of 6500 mIU/ml (First IRP) according to Romero *et al.* Using the transvaginal approach, a value of 3000 mIU/ml allows detection of normal gestational sacs including the occasional multifetal pregnancy.

In patients with minimum symptomatology or who are asymptomatic but at risk, the failure to visualize a gestational sac within the uterus with an hCG concentration in excess of these limits raises the possibility of an abnormal pregnancy and indicates the need for further evaluation. The possibility of a nonviable intrauterine pregnancy, gestational trophoblastic disease, or ectopic pregnancy should be considered.

At earlier gestations, serial hCG determinations will allow assessment of the rate of increase. In general, a normal pregnancy should exhibit at least a doubling of hCG over a 72-hour period at hCG concentrations below these limits. Ectopic pregnancies tend to demonstrate a slower rate of rise, no rise, or even a fall in hCG concentrations. Failure of an appropriate rise should raise the question of a nonviable intrauterine pregnancy or an ectopic pregnancy. Gestational trophoblastic disease is characterized by higher concentrations of hCG with unusually rapid increases in hCG concentrations.

Transvaginal ultrasound offers the potential of visualizing an ectopic pregnancy. An intra-tubal or peri-tubal hematoma creates a complex mass effect that is frequently visible. The likelihood of visualization of an ectopic pregnancy is a function of the gestational age of the pregnancy, size of the pregnancy, presence or absence of hematoma formation, and the ability to approximate the pregnancy with the transducer (Fig. 14-5).

Visualization of a complex cystic cul-de-sac mass should raise the possibility of a cul-de-sac hematoma in patients at risk. Further evaluation may disclose the presence of bleeding from a corpus luteum of pregnancy of an extrauterine pregnancy.

Although the likelihood of a coexistent intrauterine pregnancy and ectopic pregnancy is unusual, it may occur. The likelihood of the presence of this type of pregnancy (heterotopic pregnancy) has been quoted to vary between 1 : 2600 to 1 : 30,000. In general, therefore, the presence of an intrauterine pregnancy excludes the likelihood of a coexistent tubal pregnancy in the vast majority of patients.

In summary, the concentration of hCG should establish the likelihood of visualizing a normal gestational sac. An abnormal trend of hCG rise should warrant an evaluation for an abnormal pregnancy including intrauterine and extrauterine locations. The presence of abnormal sonographic findings either in the adnexa or cul-de-sac should also raise concern regarding the possibility of an extrauterine pregnancy. Occasionally, an abdominal pregnancy will be visualized in the cul-de-sac with ventral displacement of the uterine corpus.

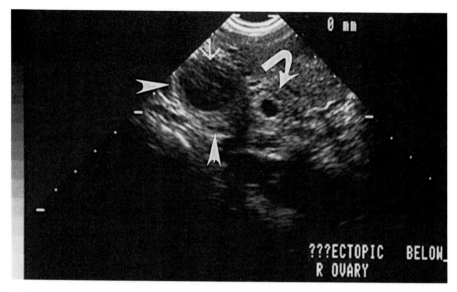

FIG. 14-5. An ectopic pregnancy *(curved arrow)* is questioned "below the R ovary." No embryonic cardiac activity could be visualized. This was an unruptured, ampullary tubal pregnancy. The ovary *(arrowheads)* exhibits a small cystic area with faint echoes suggesting a small amount of hemorrhage.

FETAL ANOMALIES

A few fetal anomalies may be diagnosed in the first trimester of pregnancy using transvaginal ultrasound. Anencephaly, cystic hygroma formation, and conjoined twins are examples of anomalous development diagnosable early in pregnancy (Figs. 14-6,14-7).

One must be cautious while attempting to diagnose fetal anomalies early in pregnancy. Occasionally, physiologic events may be construed to represent pathologic conditions. The normal anechoic appearance of the fetal brain (particularly the rhombencephalon) and the physiologic herniation of gut into the umbilical cord are both examples of these types of events. It is noteworthy that up to 30% of normal fetuses may exhibit bowel echoes in the stump of the umbilical cord at 11 weeks menstrual age (Fig. 14-8). After the first trimester, there should be no bowel echoes seen in the umbilical cord.

Some anatomical findings are associated with an increased likelihood of fetal aneuploidy. The presence of nuchal blebs, a translucent blister-like area over the fetal neck has been shown to be associated with an increased risk of aneuploidy, especially trisomy 21. A cystic hygroma, on the other hand, is more frequently associated with a monosomic X karyotype.

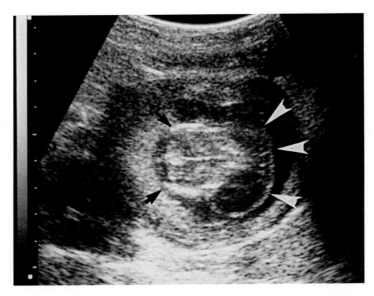

FIG. 14-6. A cystic hygroma is denoted on the posterior fetal neck *(white arrowheads)* in this first-trimester image. The parietal bony echoes are noted by the *black arrows.* Note the clearly visible midline echo of the falx cerebri.

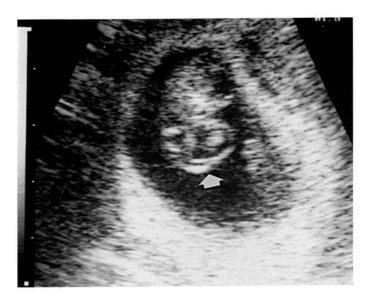

FIG. 14-7. An abnormal cephalic pole *(arrow)* is noted in this fetus at 13 weeks' gestation. The relatively hypo-echoic cerebrovasculosa characteristic of anencephaly was noted to waver on re-altime imaging.

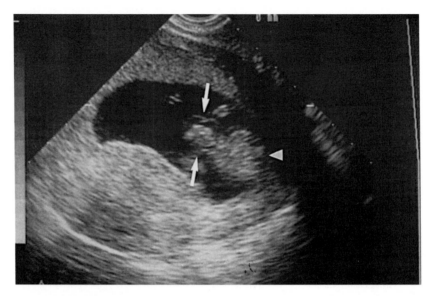

FIG. 14-8. Physiologic herniation of the gut into the proximal portion of the umbilical cord is denoted by the *large white arrows.* An axial section (cross-section) of the fetal abdomen is marked by the *white arrowhead.*

ASSOCIATED CONDITIONS

Uterine leiomyomata and ovarian cysts are the most frequently associated conditions noted in the first trimester. Leiomyomata should be measured, the location defined, and the echo pattern assessed for signs of myomatous degeneration.

Unilateral ovarian cysts frequently represent the corpus luteum of pregnancy. These resolve spontaneously near the end of the first trimester. With multifetal pregnancy, the elevated hCG concentration may produce a multicystic appearance to both ovaries. These are usually theca-lutein cysts (hyper-reactio luteinalis) and will resolve following the pregnancy.

Unilocular anechoic cysts are usually serous-type cysts and may be followed expectantly. More complex cysts may represent a cystic teratoma and warrant further diagnosis and therapy. Solid masses and potentially neoplastic masses are infrequently encountered in the first trimester. When seen, a thorough workup and evaluation is indicated. The luteoma of pregnancy will appear as a solid-type mass with dense echoes but with a significant amount of through transmission. These masses resolve following pregnancy without therapy.

SUMMARY

Realtime ultrasound, especially via the transvaginal approach, offers the potential to diagnose the presence or absence of an intrauterine pregnancy very early in gestation. In addition, the potential viability, gestation age, number of fetuses, and associated conditions may also be evaluated. The preclinical diagnosis of extrauterine pregnancy, a nonviable intrauterine pregnancy, or gestational trophoblastic disease can result in earlier, more definitive therapy and less morbidity for the patient.

FURTHER READING

Bree RL, Marn CS. Transvaginal sonography in the first trimester: embryology, anatomy, and hCG correlation. *Seminars in Ultrasound, CT, and MRI.* 1990;11:12–21.

Cadkin AV, McAlpin J. The decidua-chorionic sac: a reliable sonographic indicator of intrauterine pregnancy prior to detection of a fetal pole. *J Ultrasound Med* 1984;3:539–48.

Dickey RP, Olar TT, Taylor SN, Curole DN, Matulich EM. Relationship of small gestational sac-crown-rump length differences to abortion and abortus karyotypes. *Obstet Gynecol* 1992;79:554–7.

Frates MC, Benson CB, Doubilet PM. Pregnancy outcome after a first trimester sonogram demonstrating fetal cardiac activity. *J Ultrasound Med* 1993;12:383–6.

Kadar N, Bohrer M. Kemmann E, Shelden R. The discriminatory human chorionic gonadotropin zone for endovaginal sonography: a prospective, randomized study. *Fertil Steril* 1994;61:1016–20.

Merchiers EH, Dhont M, DeSutter PA, Beghin CJ, Vandekerckhove DA. Predictive value of early cardiac activity for pregnancy outcome. *Am J Obstet Gynecol* 1991;165:11–4.

Nyberg DA, Laing FC, Filly RA. Threatened abortion: sonographic distinction of normal and abnormal gestational sacs. *Radiology* 1986;158:397–400.

Nyberg DA, Laing FC, Filly RA, Uri-Simmons M, Jeffrey RB. Ultrasonographic differentiation of the gestational sac of early intrauterine pregnancy from the pseudogestational sac of ectopic pregnancy. *Radiology* 1983;146:755–9.

Pennell RG, Needleman L, Pajak T, Baltarowich O, Vilaro M, Goldberg BB, et al. Prospective comparison of vaginal and abdominal sonography in normal early pregnancy. *J Ultrasound Med* 1991;10:63–7.

Robinson HP, Fleming JE. A critical evaluation of sonar crown-rump length measurements. *Br J Obstet Gynaecol* 1975;82:702–10.

Romero R, Kadar N, Jeanty P, Copel JA, Chervanak FA, DeCherney A, Hobbins JC. Diagnosis of ectopic pregnancy: value of the discriminatory human chorionic gonadotropin zone. *Obstet Gynecol* 1985;66:357–60.

Timor-Tritsch IE, Farine D, Rosen MG. A close look at early embryonic development with the high frequency transvaginal transducer. *Am J Obstet Gynecol* 1988;159:676–81.

15

Evaluation of the Nonpregnant Uterus and Ovaries

The effects of estrogen stimulation on müllerian structures and the change in ovarian size and morphology as a result of ovulation and follicular estrogen production result in marked differences in the sonographic appearance of the uterus and ovaries as a function of age and hormonal status. Accurate interpretation of sonographic images mandates knowledge of the patient's physiologic status. The anatomic characteristics of normal pelvic anatomy will be discussed in the premenarchal, reproductive, and post-reproductive age groups.

PREMENARCHAL ANATOMY

Following fusion of the paired müllerian ducts, the uterus is essentially a tubular organ. The müllerian ducts form the uterus, cervix, fallopian tubes, and upper vagina. In the child, the fundus and cervix are essentially the same size. Fundal dominance is the result of estrogen stimulation of the myometrium and begins to develop concomitantly with ovarian estrogen production.

Consequently, the premenarchal uterus appears to be a small oblong structure with little sonographic difference between the fundus and cervix. The endometrial echo is usually not well defined and frequently difficult to delineate (Fig. 15-1).

If difficulty is encountered visualizing the premenarchal uterus via transabdominal scanning, one may attempt to image the lower genital tract via a transperineal approach. A linear, curvilinear, or sector transducer may be sheathed and positioned on the perineum and introitus. Depending upon the depth of resolution of the transducer, a variable amount of lower genital tract anatomy may be seen. A small amount of urine in the bladder will assist in delineating the uterus. The majority of premenarchal patients cannot tolerate a transvaginal transducer.

As noted above, the endometrium is very thin and frequently not apparent in this age group. The finding of a prominent endometrium should raise the ques-

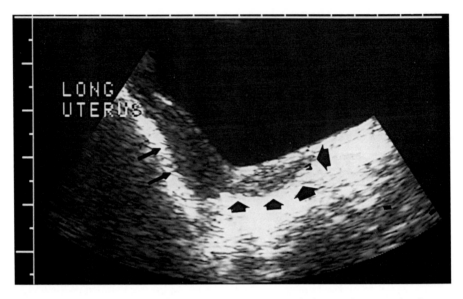

FIG. 15-1. Transabdominal longitudinal image of a premenarchal uterus demonstrating the uterine cervix (*broad arrows*) and the fundus (*narrow arrows*). Note the relative size of the fundus and cervix and the lack of fundal dominance that is seen after estrogen stimulation.

tion of exogenous ingestion of estrogen containing compounds or endogenous production of estrogen by estrogen-producing neoplasms.

Although the maximum number of germ cells are present in the ovary during fetal life, visible significant follicular activity is usually noted only in the immediate prepubertal period. The premenarchal ovary of childhood consists of predominate stroma and small follicles but these are not prominent from a sonographic standpoint. Consequently, the ultrasound appearance of the ovary is a small, predominately solid ovoid structure located lateral to the uterus. The normal premenarchal ovary is frequently difficult to visualize. Cystic ovarian masses in childhood warrant thorough investigation. In the premenarchal patient, follicular recruitment and development must be considered as potential etiologies in the evaluation of small cystic areas within the ovary.

In the neonatal period, an occasional fetal ovarian cyst may be seen. *In utero* ovarian stimulation by maternal gonadotropic hormones may produce functional ovarian cysts in the fetus. These cysts should rapidly disappear during the newborn period and, therefore, warrant expectant follow-up only.

In addition to cystic ovarian masses, the differential diagnosis of cystic adnexal masses in childhood should include cystic masses of genitourinary origin such as ureterocele or hydroureter and congenital parovarian cysts. The detection of solid adnexal masses in this age group should raise the question of ovarian stromal or germ cell tumors, enlarged lymph nodes, or other retroperitoneal neoplastic masses. Complex adnexal masses of ovarian origin must be considered to be germ cell neoplasms until proven otherwise.

REPRODUCTIVE AGE GROUP

With onset of follicular recruitment and maturation, estrogen secretion, and progesterone production, marked changes in the morphology of the uterus and ovaries are noted. In patients with gonadal dysgenesis, the administration of exogenous estrogen will produce rapid maturational changes in uterine morphology.

The fundal/cervix ratio increases dramatically. In addition to becoming larger, the fundus also becomes more bulbous in shape resulting in the uterine configuration frequently described as pear shaped. Table 15-1 depicts the size of the uterus and relationship of cervix/fundus ratio in premenarchal, reproductive, and postmenopausal patients. The endocervical canal and endometrium are readily visualized by transvaginal scanning. Measurement of the size of the uterus is usually straightforward. Most authors would suggest measuring the fundus from the internal cervical os to the top of the fundus for the sagittal longitudinal measurement. Anteroposterior and axial measurements complete the assessment of the size of the fundus.

The endometrial appearance varies predictably with the menstrual cycle. During the early proliferative phase, the endometrium appears nearly isoechoic with the myometrium (Fig. 15-2). Following estrogen-induced glandular proliferation, the endometrial surface becomes crowded with endometrial glands and, therefore, more echogenic. This results in a multilayered appearance (Fig. 15-3). In the late secretory/immediate premenstrual phase, the endometrium may appear quite echogenic due to the cellular density of the endometrium (Fig. 15-4).

The luteinization and secretory transformation during the luteal phase increases the echogenicity of the endometrial echo. The basalis layer is more echogenic than the more superficial layers. This finding is thought to be due to more water content in the functional layer of the endometrium.

TABLE 15-1. *Uterine size (in cm) and cervix-to-fundus ratio in premenarchal, reproductive, and postmenopausal women*

	Length	Width	Anteroposterior diameter	Cervix:Fundus
Reproductive	6–10	3–6	3–6	1:2
Premenopausal	3–5	2–3	2–3	4:1
Postmenopausal	3–5	2–3	2–3	1:1

From Fleischer AC, Kepple DM, Entman SS. In: Timor-Tritsch I, Rottem S, eds. *Transvaginal Sonography of Uterine Disorders in Transvaginal Sonography.* Elsevier, 2nd ed. 1991;113.

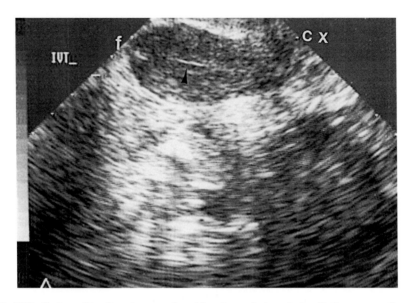

FIG. 15-2. Early proliferative phase endometrium is nearly isoechoic with the surrounding myometrium. The thin linear echo of the two adjacent endometrial surfaces (*black arrowhead*) is the most prominent sonographic finding in this patient on cycle day 6. (*f*, uterine fundus; *cx*, cervix.)

Menstrual endometrium appears less uniform in appearance. Endometrial hematoma formation is apparent. The echogenicity of the endometrium is diminished with the onset of menstrual discharge.

The serosa of the myometrium is readily defined throughout the cycle. In the secretory period, the arcuate vessels are prominent in the subserosal portion of the myometrium.

Ovarian morphology during the reproductive years is characterized by prominent follicular activity (Fig. 15-5). Periovulatory follicles approach 20 mm in size. Multiple follicles are frequently seen in the reproductive age group. The presence of follicular activity enhances the ability of the sonographer to locate the ovary in this age group.

Occasionally, cystic follicles or follicle cysts may develop. These are transient findings of normal gametogenesis and should be treated expectantly. Following ovulation the corpus luteum controls the remainder of the cycle. The corpus luteum appears as an anechoic area within the ovarian stroma. Hemorrhage into a corpus luteum will produce a small cystic area with intracystic complex echoes resulting from blood. These are also transient findings and justify expectant management.

The cervix will frequently exhibit prominent endocervical mucus around the time of ovulation and in the secretory phase. Nabothian cysts may be seen within the cervical stroma.

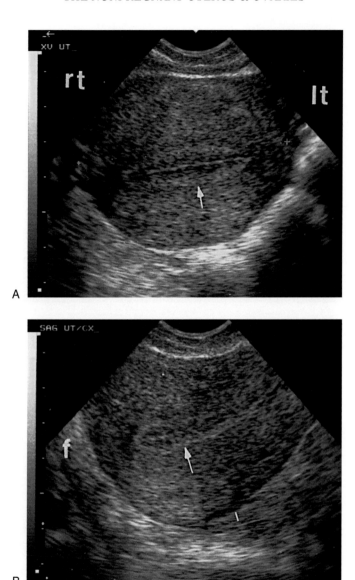

FIG. 15-3. The upper image (**A**) is oriented in the coronal plane (note *rt* and *lt*) and the lower image (**B**) is in the sagittal plane (*f*, uterine fundus). Note the multilayered appearance of the endometrium in this reproductive-age patient. The thin linear echo arising from the juxtaposition of the two endometrial surfaces is clearly seen in both images but is best demonstrated in the coronal image. The zona basalis (*arrows*) appears more echogenic than the zona functionalis at this phase of endometrial maturation.

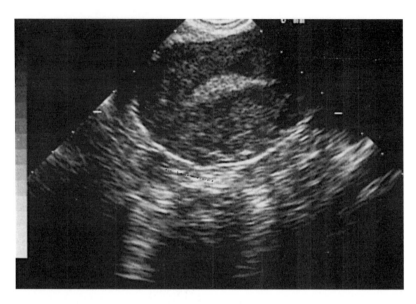

FIG. 15-4. Premenstrually, the endometrium becomes very echogenic due to the dense crowding of glands and stroma. Note the relatively echogenic appearance in this immediate premenstrual endometrium.

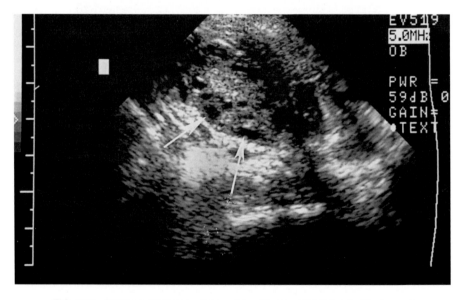

FIG. 15-5. Transvaginal image of an ovary with several follicles (*white arrows*).

POST-REPRODUCTIVE AGE GROUP

Following the cessation of ovarian function, there are marked changes in the normal anatomy of the genital tract. Obviously, ovarian changes that are frequently seen in the reproductive age group as functional processes are absent in this age group.

The uterus will diminish in size to some degree. Without estrogen stimulation, the endometrium becomes less echogenic and thinner (Fig. 15-6). Measurement of the width of the endometrial echo provides a method for assessing the presence of estrogen stimulation in this age group and is the basis for sonographic evaluation of postmenopausal bleeding.

The decrease in follicular activity makes the ovaries more difficult to delineate. Normal ovarian volume in the postmenopause should be <2.5 cm^3. This volume is calculated by the formula, volume = $d_1 \cdot d_2 \cdot d_3/2$. Occasionally, small anechoic cystic areas within the ovary are seen in this age group. If these areas are less than 5 cm, anechoic, and smooth-walled, the likelihood of malignancy is extraordinarily small.

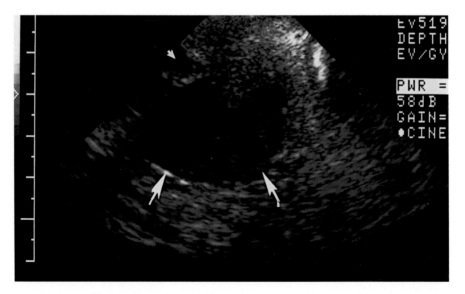

FIG. 15-6. Transvaginal longitudinal image of an anteverted uterus in a postmenopausal patient on no hormonal replacement therapy. Notice the small fundus (*large white arrows*) and poorly defined endometrial echo. The *small arrow* denotes a small amount of urine in the bladder.

SUMMARY

The appearance of genital tract anatomy is influenced by ovarian function and concomitant estrogen and progesterone stimulation. Accurate interpretation of sonographic findings of the genital tract mandates awareness of the hormonal status of the patient.

FURTHER READING

Fleischer AC, Gordon AN, Entman SS, Kepple DM. Transvaginal scanning of the endometrium. *J Clin Ultrasound* 1990;18:337–49.

16

Endometriosis and Pelvic Inflammatory Disease

Gray-scale ultrasound offers a noninvasive method for assessing the texture of pelvic masses. The ability to discern cystic from solid masses and to determine the anatomical origin of pelvic masses has enhanced the diagnostic acumen of the clinician. This chapter will focus on the ultrasound characteristics of gynecologic masses with emphasis on the utilization of vaginal sonography in patients with endometriosis and pelvic inflammatory disease. Prior to elaborating upon these specific entities, a discussion of the sonographic assessment, characterization, and classification of pelvic masses is necessary.

SONOGRAPHIC CHARACTERISTICS OF ADNEXAL MASSES

Regardless of the scanning approach, the initial assessment should determine the location and probable site of origin of the mass. In the chapter addressing scanning technique, the reader was encouraged to initiate the survey of the pelvis by locating the uterus and bladder. Once these landmarks are identified, attention is then directed to the adnexal regions.

When masses are encountered, the location should be established as either adnexal, midpelvic, or pelvo-abdominal. The site of origin is usually apparent and should be classified as either uterine, ovarian, parovarian, or nongynecologic. The presence or absence of peritoneal fluid should be noted.

Each mass should be characterized as to size and shape. Traditionally, masses are measured in three planes: cephalo-caudal, ventro-dorsal, and transverse (left–right). From these measurements the average size and/or volume may be calculated.

Following measurement of the mass and establishing the location and probable site of origin, the internal echo texture is evaluated. Totally cystic masses containing clear, serous-type fluid will appear virtually anechoic (Fig. 16-1). Low-level echo return may be seen with increasing gain settings (sensitivity) or with high protein concentration of the fluid.

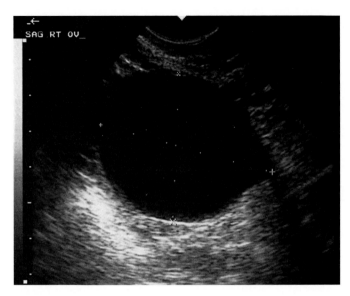

FIG. 16-1. Transvaginal image of a unilocular anechoic cyst of ovary with a smooth cyst wall and no papillations characteristic of a serous cyst. The calipers denote a cyst size of 5.2 × 4.1 cm.

Cysts containing blood or bloody fluid produce a variety of echo patterns. The endometrioma or *chocolate cyst* produces a homogeneous ground-glass appearance (Fig. 16-2 and Colorplate 1 in the color section). Frequently there is little surrounding ovarian echo. The hemorrhagic corpus luteum will frequently have some irregularity to the wall and varying echodensities depending upon how much thrombus liquefaction has occurred. Frequently, normal ovarian stroma will be seen adjacent to the corpus luteum (Fig. 16-3). Fresh bleeding may appear more echogenic due to the multitude of reflecting surfaces of intact red blood cells, but becomes hypoechoic with cell lysis and thrombus formation. As the thrombus begins to resolve, the echo pattern may become variably complex.

Solid masses attenuate the insonation beam to a greater degree than cystic masses. Posterior border echoes are more difficult to see, and the internal echostructure is more difficult to define. Uterine leiomyomata fulfill these characteristics (Fig. 16-4). With the presence of calcium, virtually all of the insonation energy can be attenuated to a point at which there is minimal, if any, echo return and shadowing will result (Fig. 16-5).

In contrast, purely cystic masses transmit sound readily. In fact, there are reverberations of sonic energy at the posterior cyst interface resulting in very dense echoes along the posterior (distal) border producing sonographic enhancement (Fig. 16-6).

The presence or absence of loculation or septations should be noted. The size (thickness) of the septations and the presence of wall irregularities (papillations) should also be noted (Fig. 16-7 and Colorplate 2).

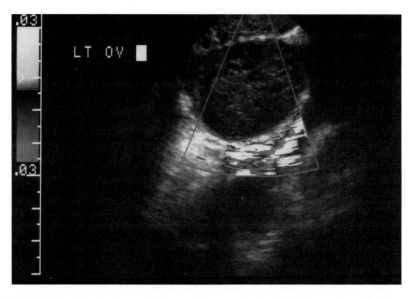

FIG. 16-2. (Colorplate 1). Ground-glass appearance of a hemorrhagic ovarian cyst. Note the small anechoic areas suggestive of early thrombus resolution.

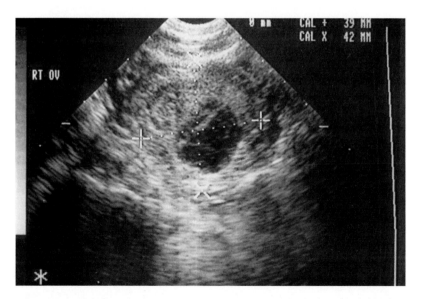

FIG. 16-3. Transvaginal image of a hemorrhagic corpus luteum of the right ovary. Notice the echogenicity suggestive of a hemorrhagic-type cyst with areas of variable echo texture.

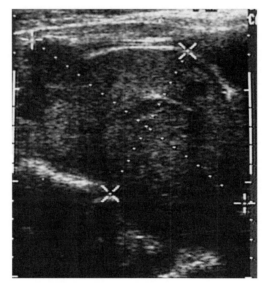

FIG. 16-4. Note the relatively poor sound transmission through this myomatous uterus. The posterior walls are difficult to delineate, confirming the solid texture of this mass.

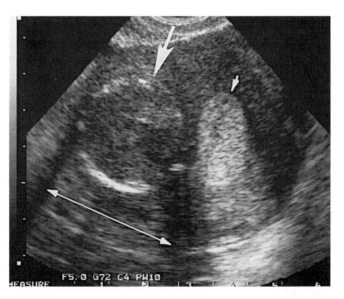

FIG. 16-5. An intramural leiomyoma with calcification (*large arrow*) is in close approximation to the endometrial echo (*small arrowhead*) on this axial transvaginal image. Note the shadowing created by the dense myoma with calcification (*thin straight arrow*) and the enhancement of the echo return produced by the endometrium.

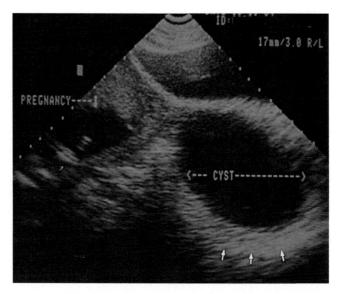

FIG. 16-6. Note the brightly echogenic area of sonic enhancement (arrow) depicting the posterior border of this purely cystic mass. This serous cyst coexisted with an intrauterine pregnancy.

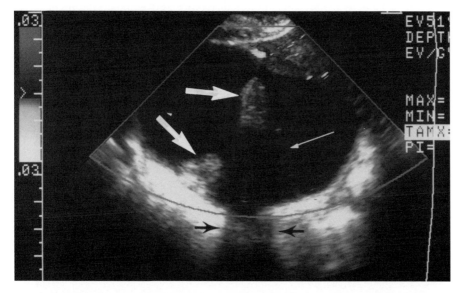

FIG. 16-7. (Colorplate 2). Transvaginal image of an ovarian cyst exhibiting thin septations (*thin arrow*) and areas of thickened epithelium between the septations and on the cyst wall (*large white arrows*). These are frequently referred to as *papillary excrescences.* Note the shadowing (*black arrows*) that results from attenuation of the sonic energy by the tissue density of the septal excrescence.

CHARACTERISTICS OF BENIGN AND MALIGNANT ADNEXAL MASSES

Masses with thick septations, irregular borders, papillations, complex disorganized echodensity, and coexistent ascites are more likely to represent a proliferative or malignant process. Those masses that are purely cystic, thinly septated (<3–4 mm or nonseptated), without papillations, and exhibiting the presence of appropriate architecture are more likely benign. Larger masses, solid masses, and those with thicker and/or irregular septations have a greater malignant potential (Figs. 16-8,16-9 and Colorplate 3). In addition, one must always remember that masses in older patients must be acknowledged to have a higher malignant potential.

The benign cystic teratoma may exhibit a range of complex echo patterns depending upon the amount of sebaceous material, serous fluid, hair, and other components that are present. The presence of calcium should alert the sonographer/sonologist of the possibility of a benign cystic teratoma (dermoid cyst) (Fig. 16-10).

Doppler sonography offers the opportunity to assess the blood flow velocity waveform from small ovarian vessels. The interpretation of Doppler waveform analysis is difficult in the reproductive years due to the marked increase in blood-flow velocity in the luteal phase. In malignant masses, there is neovascularization due to tumoral-induced angiogenesis and a resultant increase in diastolic blood-flow velocity. This results in less difference between the systolic peak ve-

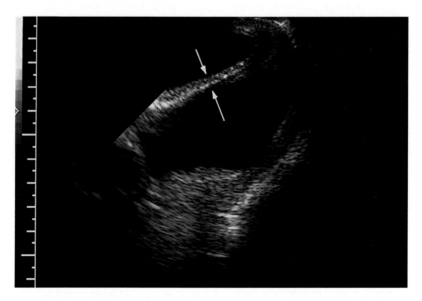

FIG. 16-8. A bilocular ovarian cyst exhibiting a thick septum (*thin arrows*).

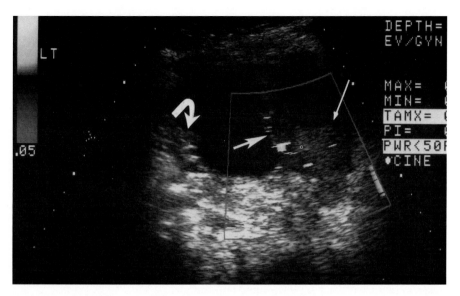

FIG. 16-9. (Colorplate 3). A cystic mass with marked tissue excrescence (*curved arrow*), thickened and vascularized septations (*arrow*), and irregular cyst wall epithelial lining (*thin arrow*) characterize this papillary serous cystadenocarcinoma of ovary.

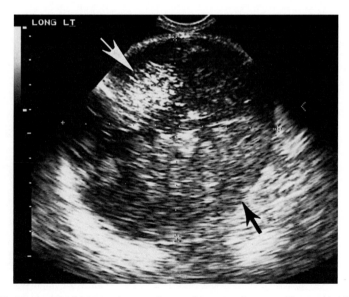

FIG. 16-10. Transvaginal image of a complex cystic mass of ovary with remarkably different echodensities. The *white arrow* represents a mass of hair and the *black arrow,* sebaceous material in a benign cystic teratoma.

locity and the diastolic nadir velocity. The waveform exhibits a narrowed or de-creased pulsatility that may be expressed as the S/D ratio, pulsatility index (S-D/Mean), or resistance index (S-D/S) (S, Systolic velocity and D, Diastolic ve-locity in cm/sec.) (Fig. 16-11 and Colorplate 4).

Many scoring systems have been developed to describe both the two-dimen-sional and Doppler findings of adnexal masses. It appears that close scrutiny of the two-dimensional image, particularly from realtime intravaginal techniques, is an accurate assessor of the origin and significance of most adnexal masses. In a review of 65 epithelial ovarian tumors and 141 benign controls, Conte *et al.* notes that ultrasound evaluation demonstrated a sensitivity of 84.7% and specificity of 92.3% in discerning benign from malignant masses. Furthermore, of 144 patients undergoing exploration for simple cysts in Vienna, only three were malignant. One of these was a tumor of low-malignant potential and all three were >7 cm in diameter.

Classification of pelvic masses into groupings based on anatomic structure and internal echo pattern seen with sonography will assist in narrowing the differen-tial diagnosis of a given adnexal mass. Table 16-1 offers a listing of likely diag-noses in masses of varying ultrasound appearances.

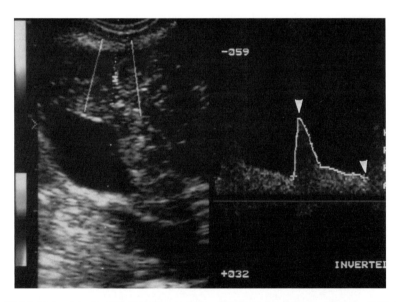

FIG. 16-11. (Colorplate 4). A Doppler flow velocity waveform of an intra-ovarian vessel. Note the sampling range gate within the ovarian stroma (*upper left*). The *left arrowhead* depicts the sys-tolic maximum velocity and the *right arrowhead,* the diastolic nadir velocity.

TABLE 16–1. *Differential diagnosis of cystic adnexal masses*

Structure	Internal echodensity	Dx possibilities
Unilocular	Anechoic/hypoechoic	Follicle/cystic follicle
		Serous cyst
		Parovarian cyst
		Hydrosalpinx
Multilocular	Anechoic/hypoechoic	Multiple follicles
		Serous cystadenoma
		Mucinous cystadenoma
Unilocular	Uniform echogenicity	Hemorrhagic cyst
	Ground-glass appearance	Endometrioma
		Corpus hemorrhagicum
Unilocular	Variable echogenicity	Corpus hemorrhagicum
Multilocular	Variable echodensity	Endometrioma
		Inflammatory complex
Unilocular	Variable solid/cystic	Teratoma
		Inflammatory complex
		Carcinoma
Multilocular	Variable solid/cystic	Carcinoma
		Benign neoplasms

ENDOMETRIOSIS

Neither transabdominal nor transvaginal ultrasound evaluation establishes the diagnosis of endometriosis. Scattered, peritoneal-surface, endometriotic implants are rarely visible by ultrasound scanning techniques. Many of these patients will have an increased amount of peritoneal fluid but not overt ascites. Occasionally, a large implant in the cul-de-sac of Douglas may be visible via transvaginal scanning.

Endometriosis produces a spectrum of sonographic findings that is commensurate with the amount of bleeding, degree of thrombus formation/resolution, and the amount of adhesive disease. Extensive bowel adhesions may significantly compromise definitive image characterization of an endometriotic mass due to the presence of intraluminal bowel gas that impedes transmission of the insonation energy.

The visualization of cystic, polycystic, septated, and irregular masses was reported using static, grayscale sonography in the late 1970s. The predictive capability of ultrasound in the diagnosis of endometriosis was assessed by Friedman *et al.* in 1985. They reported that, in a series of 85 patients, ultrasound correctly diagnosed endometriosis in 4 of 37 patients (10.8%). Therefore, ultrasound does not appear to offer the clinician the ability to screen patients for endometriosis.

Nonetheless, characterization of palpable masses by ultrasound may increase or decrease clinical suspicion of endometriosis. The finding of unilateral or bilateral cysts of the ovary with a homogeneous, ground-glass internal echodensity certainly is highly suggestive of ovarian endometrioma formation (Fig. 16-12).

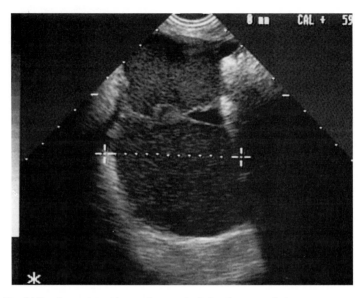

FIG. 16-12. A bilocular endometrioma of ovary depicting the ground-glass appearance of an intracystic, chocolate-cyst fluid.

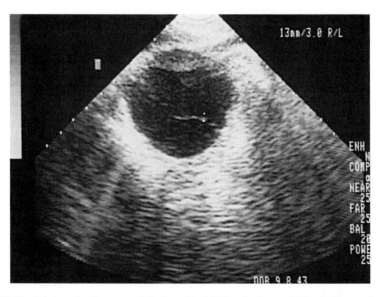

FIG. 16-13. A hemorrhagic corpus luteal cyst exhibiting features similar to those of an endometrioma.

The differentiation from hemorrhagic corpora lutea frequently requires a repeat study following a menstrual cycle or two (Fig. 16-13).

PELVIC INFLAMMATORY DISEASE

Pelvic inflammatory disease is a polymicrobial infection of the genital tract most commonly affecting the uterus, fallopian tubes, and ovaries. Common pathogens include *Neisseria gonorrhea* and *Chlamydia trachomatis*. The resultant adhesive disease, oophoritis, and occasional abscess formation produce a variety of sonographic findings. The majority of patients with acute salpingitis may exhibit normal ultrasound findings.

In contrast to acute salpingitis, chronic pelvic inflammatory disease results in the formation of hydrosalpinges, tubo-ovarian complexes, and bowel adhesions. Hydrosalpinx formation results from agglutination of the tubal fimbria and resultant accumulation of intra-tubal fluid. Hydrosalpinges appear as elongated, hypo-echoic areas juxtaposed to the ovary (Fig. 16-14). The presence of intraluminal bowel gas in adhered loops of bowel may decrease the acuity of the image in these patients. In addition, inflammatory conditions of the pelvis may produce mural thickening of the gut thereby changing its sonographic appearance to some degree.

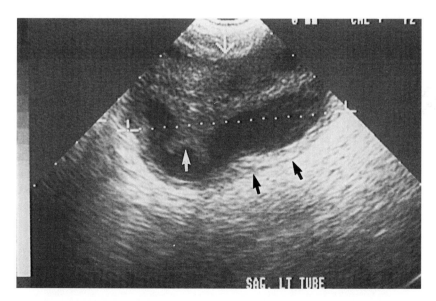

FIG. 16-14. This elongated tubular structure is a chronic hydrosalpinx. Note the intratubal papillations (*small white arrow*) and thickened inferior tubal wall (*black arrow*). The length of this hydrosalpinx is denoted by the calipers to be 72 mm. The superior echo (*larger white arrow*) denoted the remainder of a tubo-ovarian inflammatory complex. No abscess formation is seen in this image.

The inflamed ovary may exhibit prominent stromal echoes, and the existing follicles will appear more prominent (Fig. 16-15). Adhesions around the ovary and/or between the ovary and the fallopian tube create a tubo-ovarian complex. This structure appears irregular, variably complex, and frequently difficult to delineate precisely due to ultrasonic interference from intraluminal bowel gas.

Occasionally, a tubo-ovarian abscess or pelvic abscess will result (Fig. 16-16). These masses exhibit the thickened walls, intracystic echogenicity characteristic of purulent fluid, and frequent septations. Ultrasound guidance enhances the clinician's ability to drain/aspirate these abscesses thereby improving the patient's response to antibiotic therapy.

In contrast to endometriosis, endovaginal sonography appears to perform well as a diagnostic tool in the patient with pelvic inflammatory disease. In a small study of 16 patients who underwent laparoscopy following endovaginal ultrasound examination, Patten et al. noted a sensitivity of 91% and a specificity of 93% on the prediction of tubal or peri-tubal disease.

The response of patients to antibiotic therapy may be monitored by serial ultrasound scanning. The utilization of ultrasound for this purpose will be discussed later.

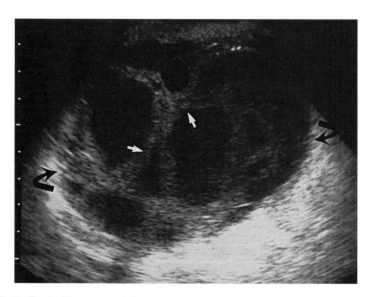

FIG. 16-15. Oophoritis may result in prominent ovarian stromal echoes (*white arrows*) surrounding intraovarian follicles as noted in this image of an ovary (*curved black arrows*) in a patient with acute salpingo-oophoritis.

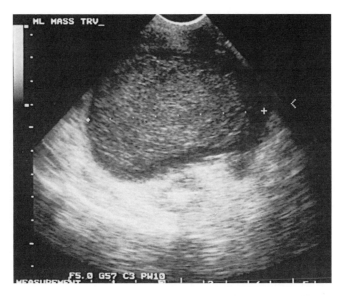

FIG. 16-16. This echogenic cul-de-sac mass represents a pelvic abscess with an extensive accumulation of purulent material. The calipers delineate that this abscess is 7.8 cm in transverse diameter.

SUMMARY

Gray-scale ultrasound scanning offers the sonographer/sonologist the opportunity to define the anatomic location, site of origin, and internal echo characterization of pelvic masses. Using abdominal or endovaginal realtime techniques, the clinician has access to potentially valuable information regarding the gross anatomical characteristics of the existing pathology.

Controversy exists regarding the appropriate use of ultrasound in these patients. Most would agree, however, that if the potential information that may be gained could alter the patient's management, then it is worthwhile to perform the study. With this in mind, it appears that the use of ultrasound for the patient with suspected endometriosis or pelvic inflammatory disease as an extension to and enhancement of the pelvic examination is appropriate.

The ability to expand or contract a differential diagnosis of a pelvic mass or of a patient's symptomatology will allow more precise and individualized care. In addition, if other parameters offer confusing or indeterminant evidence of response to therapy, serial imaging may offer a more objective measure of the adequacy of treatment.

FURTHER READING

Cacciatore B, Leminen A, Ingman-Friberg S, *et al*. Transvaginal sonographic findings in ambulatory patients with suspected pelvic inflammatory disease. *Obstet Gynecol* 1992:80:912–6.

Conte M, Guariglia L, Benedetti P, *et al*. Ovarian carcinoma: an ultrasound study. *Eur J Gynaecol Oncol* 1990;11:33–6.

Friedman H, Vogelzang RL, Mendelson EB, *et al*. Endometriosis detection by ultrasound with laparoscopic correlation. *Radiology* 1985;157:217–20.

Obwegeser R, Deutinger J, Bernascheck G. The risk of malignancy with an apparently simple adnexal cyst on ultrasound. *Arch Gynecol Obstet* 1993;253:117–20.

Patten RM, Vincent LM, Wolner-Hanssen P, *et al*. Pelvic inflammatory disease. Endovaginal sonography with laparoscopic correlation. *J Ultrasound Med* 1990;9:681–9.

Sandler MA, Karo JJ. The spectrum of ultrasonic findings in endometriosis. *Radiology* 1978;127:229–31.

Walsh JW, Taylor KJ, Rosenfield AT. Gray scale ultrasonography in the diagnosis of endometriosis and adenomyosis. *Am J Roentgenol* 1979;132:87–90.

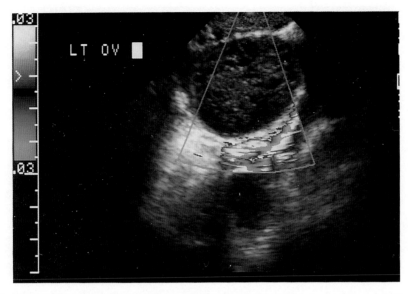

Colorplate 1. (Fig. 16-2). Ground-glass appearance of a hemorrhagic ovarian cyst. Note the small anechoic areas suggestive of early thrombus resolution.

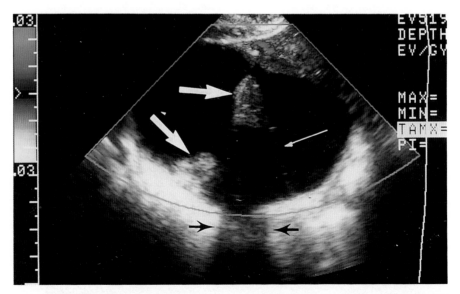

Colorplate 2. (Fig. 16-7). Transvaginal image of an ovarian cyst exhibiting thin septations *(thin arrow)* and areas of thickened epithelium between the septations and on the cyst wall *(large white arrows)*. These are frequently referred to as papillary excrescences. Note the shadowing *(black arrows)* that results from attenuation of the sonic energy by the tissue density of the septal excrescence.

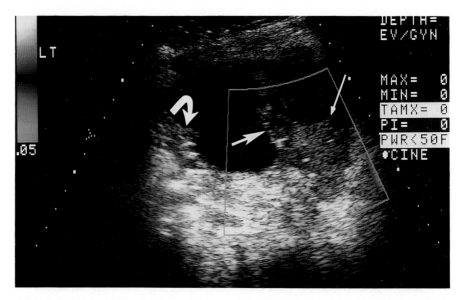

Colorplate 3. (Fig. 16-9). A cystic mass with marked tissue excrescence *(curved arrow)*, thickened and vascularized septations *(arrowhead)*, and irregular cyst wall epithelial lining *(thin arrow)* characterize this papillary serous cystadenocarcinoma of ovary.

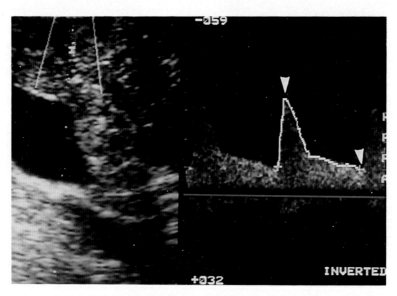

Colorplate 4. (Fig. 16-11). A Doppler flow velocity waveform of an intraovarian vessel. Note the sampling range gate within the ovarian stroma *(upper left)*. The *left arrowhead* depicts the systolic maximum velocity and the *right arrowhead* the diastolic nadir velocity.

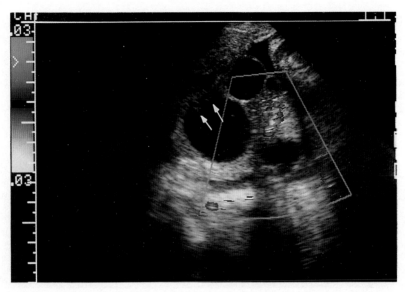

Colorplate 5. (Fig. 17-6). This ovarian cyst is multilocular, complex, highly vascular, and exhibits papillary excrescences on the cyst wall. All of these characteristics suggest malignancy. This represents a serous adenocarcinoma of the ovary.

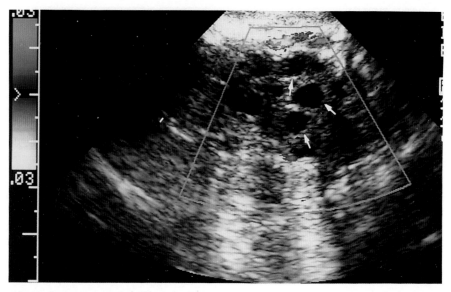

Colorplate 6. (Fig. 18-1). Multiple small follicles are delineated by the *arrow* in this patient beginning a cycle of clomiphene citrate for ovulation induction.

17

Perimenopausal and Postmenopausal Screening of Ovary and Endometrium for Neoplastic Disease

Gynecologic malignancy contributes to the morbidity and mortality of the older gynecologic patient. Whereas screening programs for the detection of cervical dysplasia have resulted in a marked decrease in the frequency of cervical carcinoma, the same cannot be said for malignancies of the endometrium and ovary. This chapter will address the current status of endovaginal sonography in the early diagnosis of these two malignancies. The advantages and disadvantages of sonographic screening for these malignancies will also be discussed. Throughout this chapter, the reader must be aware of the difference between case detection and population screening by ultrasonographic techniques.

ENDOMETRIAL CARCINOMA

Patients with adenocarcinoma of the endometrium typically present with abnormal uterine bleeding. Many of these patients have had unopposed estrogenic stimulation of the endometrium and pre-existing hyperplasia of the endometrium.

The normal sonographic appearance of the endometrium was described in the chapter addressing normal gynecologic anatomy. Following the menopause, the endogenous stimulation of the endometrium by follicular estrogen declines. Consequently, both the thickness and echogenicity of the endometrium decrease.

The thickness of the endometrium may be assessed in several ways. Many would suggest measurement of the endometrial single-layer thickness. Others prefer the total width of the thickest portion of the fundal endometrium (Fig. 17-1). Unless otherwise stated, endometrial thickness in this chapter will refer to total width or double-layer thickness.

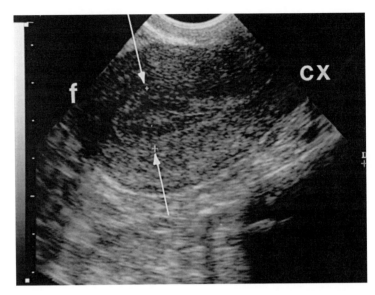

FIG. 17-1. Measurement of the thickness of the endometrium. This is a double-layer thickness measurement from the basalis/myometrial interface on one side to the other (*long arrows*). The calipers indicate that this reproductive age patient has an endometrial thickness of 16 mm. Uterine fundus labeled (*f*) and cervix is (*cx*).

In postmenopausal patients with abnormal uterine bleeding, an endometrial thickness (double layer) <5 mm has not been associated with endometrial adenocarcinoma. In a study of 1000 women undergoing endovaginal ultrasound and endometrial sampling, Wikland noted that the mean endometrial thickness of those patients with adenocarcinoma was 18 mm (5–55 mm). In these patients, there has not been a diagnosis of endometrial cancer with a double-layer thickness ≤4 mm. The average thickness of patients with endometrial hyperplasia was noted to be 10 mm (6–13 mm) (Fig. 17-2).

Therefore, in postmenopausal patients who are not on hormonal replacement therapy, an endometrial thickness of <5 mm is very reassuring. A thickness of >10 mm suggests possible endometrial hyperplasia and justifies sampling for histologic study.

Patients who exhibit an endometrial thickness >5 mm, but <10 mm are in the borderline group. Their management must be individualized based upon other historical and physical findings.

Due to the relatively low prevalence of endometrial adenocarcinoma, population screening by endovaginal sonography does not appear feasible. For patients with abnormal uterine bleeding or for those at increased risk, endovaginal evaluation of the endometrial thickness may heighten or lessen concern about a proliferative endometrial process.

For patients on hormonal replacement therapy, the normal limits for endometrial thickness are less clearly defined. In a group of 30 women on cyclic estro-

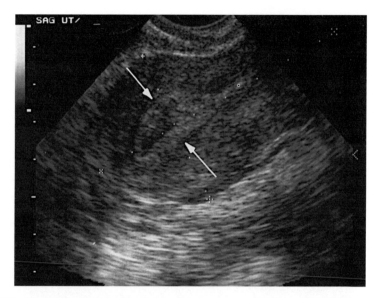

FIG. 17-2. Transvaginal image of an anteverted uterus measuring 7.5 × 4.2 cm through the fundus with an abnormal endometrial thickness of 13 mm (*long arrows*) in a patient with complex endometrial hyperplasia without atypia.

gen with progesterone added for the last 10 days of a 21-day cycle, 5 patients (17%) had endometrial double-layer thickness >5 mm compared with only 15.5% of the control group not on hormonal replacement therapy.

Lin *et al.* studied 112 patients, of whom 54 were receiving hormonal replacement therapy and 58 were not. The mean (± SD) endometrial thickness of the patients on unopposed estrogen or sequential estrogen and progesterone was 6.8 mm (±5.3 mm) and 6.6 mm (±3.9 mm), respectively. Those on combined estrogen and progesterone had a mean (±SD) thickness of 5.3 mm (±1.7 mm) and those on no therapy exhibited a thickness of 5.2 mm (±4.5 mm).

In practice, therefore, one must consider the type of hormonal replacement therapy the patient is taking when interpreting the significance of an endometrial thickness measurement. Data to support this recommendation are accumulating but are not yet firmly established.

Occasionally, the endometrium will exhibit a small fluid collection. Although most studies do not reveal an association of endometrial fluid with endometrial carcinoma, this finding has been associated with occult gynecologic malignancy of other sites including cervix (hematometria/pyometria) and, rarely, carcinoma of the ovary. The likelihood of an occult cancer is apparently very low. Goldstein reported in a series of 30 patients with endometrial fluid collections that, in patients with an endometrial thickness ≤3 mm, endometrial sampling is unnecessary. If the endometrial thickness is >3 mm (single layer) or 6 mm (double layer), then endometrial sampling is justified.

Endometrial polyps may also be seen. Polyps are usually more echogenic than is the surrounding endometrium. If associated with surrounding endometrial fluid, they will appear more echogenic and more apparent. If in doubt, a small amount of sterile fluid (saline) may be instilled to more clearly outline intrauterine anatomy. This technique is referred to as *hysterosonography* (Fig. 17-3).

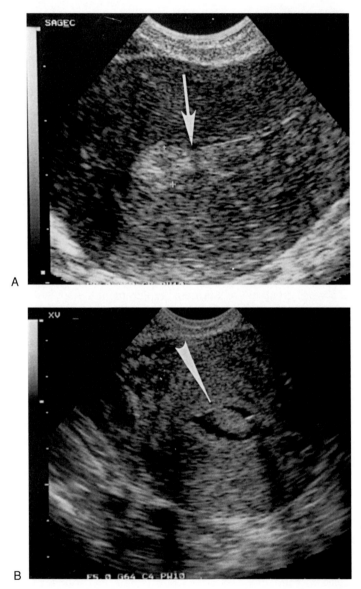

FIG. 17-3. A,B: An endometrial polyp (*arrow*) was questioned in this patient with abnormal uterine bleeding. Infusion of saline into the endometrial cavity clearly delineates a small fundal polyp.

Submucous leiomyomata are readily visualized by endovaginal sonography. These appear to distort the endometrial echo to varying degrees and exhibit the solid characteristics of a leiomyoma (Fig. 17-4).

The role of endovaginal ultrasound in the assessment of the patient with peri-

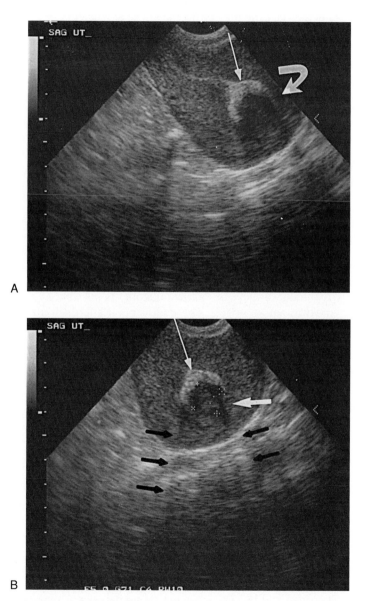

FIG. 17-4. The upper image (A) is in the sagittal plane, the lower image (B) is oriented coronally. A small submucous myoma (*large white arrows*) measuring 1.5 × 1.4 cm distorts the endometrial cavity (*thin white arrows*). Although relatively hypoechoic, note the shadowing (*small black arrows*) that results from this myoma confirming its solid nature.

menopausal or postmenopausal bleeding is essentially one of evaluating the gross anatomic intrauterine anatomy that exists. Bleeding from an atrophic endometrium is not an uncommon finding. These patients have a very thin endometrial echo.

Likewise, the patient with a modest amount of abnormal bleeding that exhibits a prominent endometrial echo may be deemed to be at greater risk and, therefore, justify a more aggressive sampling approach.

OVARIAN CARCINOMA

Approximately 24,000 American women were estimated to have developed ovarian carcinoma in 1994. Unfortunately, the majority of these patients have advanced-stage disease at the time of diagnosis and, therefore, approximately 13,699 deaths will occur as a result of this disease. The mortality rate for ovarian cancer has changed little over the past 30 years. At the present time, research continues to evaluate a multimodal approach to allow screening of the at-risk population for this malignancy.

The use of serum, tumor-associated antigens as an initial screen is controversial. A significant number of early stage cancers do not exhibit elevation of these antigens, and an elevated antigen concentration is frequently not due to an occult malignancy. The positive predictive value of an elevated antigen is extremely low, and the false-positive rate is high.

Ultrasonographic assessment of ovarian anatomy is possible by the transabdominal or transvaginal approach. The endovaginal approach allows an enhanced image and allows more precise definition of intraovarian architecture.

As noted earlier in this text, malignant ovarian masses tend to exhibit a complex echo structure with cystic and solid components with disorganized architecture. Thick septations and/or papillary excrescences are seen frequently. Solid ovarian masses have a greater malignant potential than purely cystic lesions.

Using transabdominal ultrasound, Campbell *et al.* screened 5,479 patients at 18-month intervals for a total of 15,977 scans. Even though the odds of detecting a cancer was 1 in 67 abnormal scans, no Stage I and only 2 Stage II cancers of the ovary were detected. Four Stage II and IV tumors were diagnosed.

Using endovaginal ultrasound scanning, van Nagell *et al.* detected two Stage I ovarian cancers in 1300 asymptomatic postmenopausal patients at the University of Kentucky. Of interest, both of these patients had a normal CA-125 and pelvic examination.

Obviously, with an annual incidence of 20,000 cases, an extremely large number of asymptomatic women would have to be screened annually to detect patients with Stage I disease. In an attempt to estimate the cost of national screening of the at-risk population by serum tumor-associated antigen (CA-125) and ultrasound, Creasman and DiSaia estimated an annual cost of over $13 billion. They also point out that there are no data to suggest that this effort would necessarily result in a decreased mortality rate.

Because mass screening with either tumor-associated antigens and/or ultrasound does not appear to be feasible, emphasis is being placed on the evaluation of high-risk groups. Patients with a family history of ovarian cancer, other genetic predisposing states, and those with palpable masses may benefit from evaluation via endovaginal ultrasound.

Two-dimensional ultrasound scanning with or without color Doppler imaging provides a reliable means for evaluating internal morphology of adnexal masses. Jain evaluated 50 adnexal masses with endovaginal ultrasound in an attempt to predict malignancy versus benignancy. Using two-dimensional structural criteria similar to that mentioned above, 38 of 40 benign masses were correctly identified (Figs. 17-5,17-6 and Colorplate 5). All nine malignant masses were also identified. Two-dimensional imaging exhibited a sensitivity of 90% and specificity of 95%. The addition of color Doppler scanning did not increase the accuracy of diagnosis. Color Doppler imaging alone did not perform as well as two-dimensional ultrasound alone.

Other authors have published similar results. Physiologic events relative to ovarian physiology and variable metabolic activity of different types of adnexal masses result in similar blood flow velocity patterns. Consequently, there is an overlap of descriptive indices between the benign and malignant tumors. Secondly, since malignant masses exhibit distorted architecture, the addition of an abnormal Doppler waveform does little to increase concern.

It was hoped that abnormal Doppler flow velocity waveforms in benign-ap-

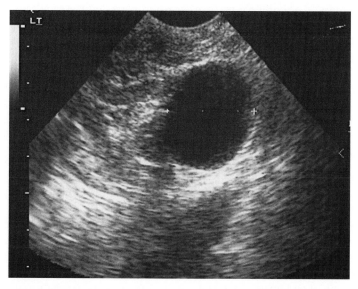

FIG. 17-5. This small (2.5 cm) unilocular anechoic ovarian cyst appears totally benign. The absence of thick septa, papillary excrescences, complex intracystic echoes, and smooth lining all suggest a benign ovarian cyst.

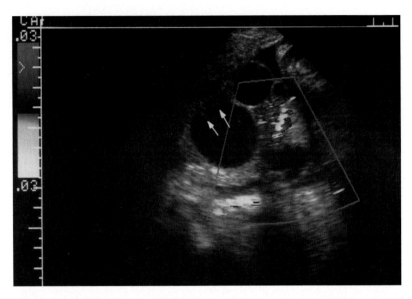

FIG. 17-6. (Colorplate 5). This ovarian cyst is multilocular, complex, highly vascular, and exhibits papillary excrescences on the cyst wall. All of these characteristics suggest malignancy. This represents a serous adenocarcinoma of the ovary.

pearing masses would allow the detection of occult malignancy. To date, this capability has not been unequivocally established.

In summary, the morphologic assessment of adnexal masses allows the clinician to predict the likelihood of malignancy with a high degree of certainty. This knowledge could allow more precise preoperative evaluation, surgical management planning, and operative management of patients with palpable adnexal masses.

The utilization of endovaginal ultrasound to screen *high-risk* populations for the presence of occult ovarian cancer appears to be justified if one accepts the relatively low positive-predictive value of the method. At the present time, there does not appear to be a reliable, cost-effective modality to allow screening of the population for the presence of occult carcinoma of the ovary.

SUMMARY

Realtime ultrasound by either the abdominal or vaginal approach offers the sonologist/sonographer the opportunity to assess the internal morphology of the uterus and ovaries. The endovaginal approach allows improved resolution albeit at the expense of depth of focus.

Evaluation of endometrial thickness in postmenopausal patients may either increase or decrease concern regarding the possibility of endometrial hyperplasia/carcinoma. The ability to discern those patients with thin endometria compatible with endometrial atrophy from those with thickened endometria compatible with endometrial hyperplasia or neoplasia allows more specific planning of the extent and type of endometrial sampling.

Endovaginal ultrasound also allows accurate definition of the internal morphology of adnexal masses. The addition of color Doppler imaging appears to add little to the accuracy of diagnosis when compared with two-dimensional imaging alone. Although endovaginal ultrasound appears to be very accurate in assessing the palpable adnexal mass, this modality alone or in combination with tumor-associated antigen sampling does not appear to offer a practical, cost-effective method of ovarian cancer screening for the entire population.

FURTHER READING

Bourne TH, Reynolds K, Campbell S. Ovarian cancer screening. *Curr Opin Radiol* 1991;3:216–24.

Campbell S, Bhan V, Royston P, *et al*. Transabdominal ultrasound screening for early ovarian cancer. *BMJ* 1989;229:1363–7.

Carlsson J, Arger P, Thompson S, *et al*. Clinical and pathologic correlation of endometrial cavity fluid detected by ultrasound in the postmenopausal patient. *Obstet Gynecol* 1991;77:119–23.

Chan FY, Chau MT, Pun TC, *et al*. Limitations of transvaginal sonography and color Doppler imaging in the differentiation of endometrial carcinoma from benign endometrial lesions. *J Ultrasound Med* 1994; 13:623–6.

Creasman WT, DiSaia PJ. Screening in ovarian cancer. *Am J Obstet Gynecol* 1991;165:7–10.

Goldstein SR, Nachtigall M, Snyder RJ, *et al*. Endometrial assessment by vaginal ultrasonography before endometrial sampling in patients with postmenopausal bleeding. *Am J Obstet Gynecol* 1990;163: 119–23.

Goldstein SR. Postmenopausal endometrial fluid collections revisited: look at the doughnut rather than the hole. *Obstet Gynecol* 1994;83:738–40.

Granberg S, Wikland M, Norstrom A. Endometrial thickness as measured by endovaginal ultrasound for identifying endometrial abnormality. *Am J Obstet Gynecol* 1991;164:47–52.

Jain KA. Prospective evaluation of adnexal masses with endovaginal gray-scale and duplex and color Doppler US: correlation with pathologic findings. *Radiology* 1994;191:63–7.

Lin MC, Gosink BB, Wolf SI, *et al*. Endometrial thickness after menopause: effect of hormone replacement. *Radiology* 1991;180:427–32.

National Institutes of Health Consensus Development Conference Statement. *Ovarian Cancer: Screening, Treatment, and Follow-up*. April 5–7, 1994.

Van-Nagell JR, DePriest PD, Puls LE, *et al*. Ovarian cancer screening in asymptomatic postmenopausal women by transvaginal sonography. *Cancer* 1991;68:458–62.

Wikland M, Granberg S, Karlsson B, *et al*. Assessment of the endometrium in the postmenopausal woman by vaginal sonography. *Ultrasound Q* 1992;10:15–27.

18

Complementary Applications in Gynecology: Ovulation Induction and Guided Procedures

OVULATION INDUCTION

A variety of pharmacologic agents are available for ovulation induction. The most commonly utilized agent is clomiphene citrate, which is thought to enhance gonadotropin stimulation of the ovary due to its action at the estrogen feedback receptor. In addition, there are gonadotropin preparations that directly stimulate follicular development.

Regardless of the method of follicular stimulation used, sonographic technology allows assessment of both follicular size and number. This information can be correlated with the serum estradiol concentration. Using this information, the likelihood of a successful ovulation induction with minimal risk of multifetal pregnancy is enhanced. The majority of patients who undergo sonographic follicular monitoring during ovulation induction are receiving gonadotropin therapy. In certain instances, sonographic assessment of follicular status may also be of benefit in those patients receiving clomiphene citrate.

In addition, evaluation of follicular status prior to a stimulation cycle will also assist in the appropriate use of these hormonal preparations and minimize the likelihood of ovarian hyperstimulation. In the unlikely event of ovarian hyperstimulation, ultrasound monitoring of ovarian size will assist in the expectant management of these patients.

With the advent of assisted reproductive techniques, including *in vitro* fertilization, gamete intra-fallopian transfer, and zygote intra-fallopian transfer, ultrasound information of follicular status and endometrial morphology has become even more important to the reproductive endocrinologist. Although discussion of specific protocols for ovulation induction and assisted reproductive technologies are beyond the scope of this chapter, the technique of follicular monitoring will be presented.

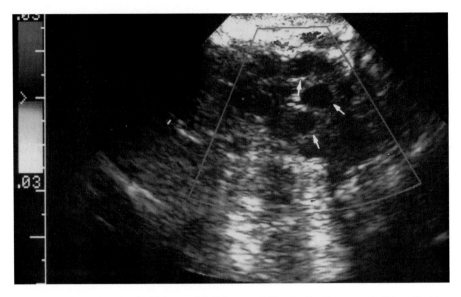

FIG. 18-1. (Colorplate 6). Multiple small follicles are delineated by the *arrow* in this patient beginning a cycle of clomiphene citrate for ovulation induction.

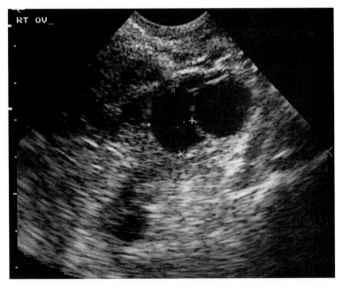

FIG. 18-2. Two follicles are seen in this image. The calipers depict that one of the follicles is 12 × 17 mm.

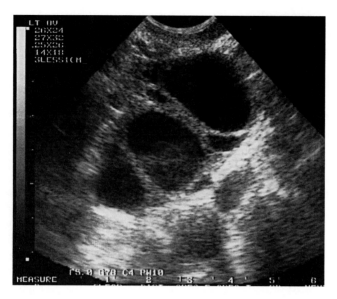

FIG. 18-3. Multiple large follicles in excess of 25 mm diameter are noted in this image.

Utilizing intravaginal scanning techniques previously described, the ovary is located in either the right or left adnexa. A 5 MHz or 7 MHz transducer will allow detailed ovarian study in the majority of patients. The higher frequency transducer will provide enhanced resolution at the expense of depth of focus.

Follicular measurements are made in three planes, and the average diameter is used to assess follicular size (Fig. 18-1 and Colorplate 6). Peri-ovulatory follicles are in the 18–22 mm range (Fig. 18-2). If follicles exceed 25 mm, they would be referred to as *follicle cysts*. Persistent follicles of 20 mm or greater range following an unsuccessful cycle are cause for concern with subsequent stimulation and should be evaluated closely prior to repeat stimulation in an effort to avoid hyperstimulation (Fig. 18-3).

Following ovulation, the corpus luteum can be visualized. Occasionally, a small amount of hemorrhage into the corpus luteum (corpus hemorrhagicum) may produce some intracystic echoes of varying echodensities.

GUIDED PROCEDURES

Transvaginal ultrasonography allows accurate guidance of needle aspiration procedures by using the tracking technology of the scanning equipment. Whereas many variations exist among manufacturers, the basic technique involves attaching a guide to the sheathed transvaginal transducer. Guides of various diameters are available. Activation of the tracking guide on the machine will project a linear track on the monitor.

By varying the angulation of the transducer, the tracking guide can be aligned with the area to be sampled. By inserting the needle along this line, a variety of aspiration procedures can be accomplished with precision. Care must be taken to prevent the vaginal apex from being pushed away from the scanning probe during needle insertion. If this occurs, the image will be degraded or even lost. Firm steady pressure will allow approximation of the scanning tip to the vaginal apex.

As the needle tip touches the vaginal apex, the operator should reassess the track guide on the monitor. With steady pressure on the transducer, the needle should be advanced without hesitation into the sampling site. The needle will be seen traversing the track guide on the monitor (Fig. 18-4).

Aspiration of cul-de-sac fluid collections, oocyte retrieval for assisted reproductive techniques, and aspiration of selected ovarian cysts are all possible utilizing this technique. Although oocyte retrieval techniques are beyond the scope of this text, suffice it to say that the necessity of a larger diameter needle and multiple aspiration attempts result in a greater likelihood that some sedation will be necessary. Simple aspirations with smaller needles (18–20 g) are readily accomplished with topical lidocaine and, at most, an oral anxiolytic medication.

The selection of patients for ultrasound-directed ovarian cyst aspiration is controversial. In order to avoid the potential of aspirating a malignant cyst, it is advisable to limit this procedure to those cysts that are at minimal risk of malignancy based upon two-dimensional ultrasound parameters. Many operators would also prefer a normal serum CA-125 prior to the procedure. Following as-

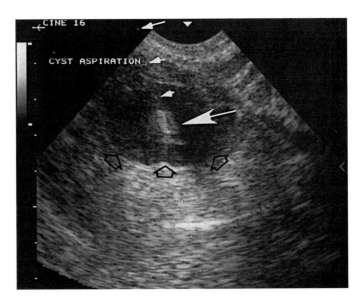

FIG. 18-4. Transvaginal image obtained during a cyst aspiration. The needle tracks are denoted by the *small arrows*. The aspiration needle is marked by a *large white arrow*. The collapsing cyst wall is designated by the *open black arrowheads*.

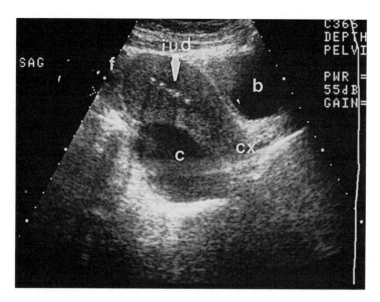

FIG. 18-5. Transabdominal sagittal image denoting the intrauterine location of a Lippes Loop IUD. Note the characteristic shadowing that results from acoustic impedance from the plastic of the IUD insonated in cross-section. There is an incidental ovarian cyst noted in the cul-de-sac (*c*). The urinary bladder is denoted by (*b*). Uterine fundus is (*f*), cervix is (*cx*).

piration, a repeat scan is suggested because of the possibility of recurrence.

Other gynecologic procedures are amenable to sonographic direction. Using the transabdominal approach, one can easily monitor the appropriate placement or removal of an intrauterine contraceptive device (Fig. 18-5). Endometrial sampling procedures and uterine curettage are also easily monitored by this technique. A moderate amount of urine to create a sonographic "window" will often facilitate these efforts. The amount of urine necessary to improve the sonographic guidance will vary with the habitus of the patient, the orientation of the uterus, and the procedure being attempted.

SUMMARY

Transvaginal and transabdominal ultrasound techniques offer the gynecologist the ability to perform a variety of complementary gynecologic procedures. The potential to visualize follicular development during ovulation induction and correlating size and number of follicles with serum estradiol levels will enhance the success of ovulation induction and lessen the likelihood of multifetal pregnancy.

Ultrasound guidance of gynecologic aspiration procedures is readily accomplished with transvaginal sonography utilizing the needle or aspiration guidance capability discussed above. Intrauterine procedures can be visualized by the transabdominal approach.

FURTHER READING

Bret PM, Guibaud L, Atri M, *et al*. Transvaginal US-guided aspiration of ovarian cysts and solid pelvic masses. *Radiology* 1992:185:377–80.

Hull ME, Moghissi KS, Magyar DM, *et al*. Correlation of serum estradiol levels and ultrasound monitoring to assess follicular maturation. *Fertil Steril* 1986;46:42–5.

Ron ER, Herman A, Weinraub Z, *et al*. Clear ovarian cyst aspiration guided by vaginal ultrasonography. *Eur J Obstet Gynecol Reprod Biol* 1991;42:43–7.

Tulandi T, Hamilton EF, Arronet GH, *et al*. Ovulation induction by human menopausal gonadotropin with ultrasonic monitoring of the ovarian follicles. *Int J Fertil* 1987;32:312–5.

19

The Office Practice

The incorporation of obstetric and gynecologic ultrasound into a busy practice, as with any new procedure, requires a careful and rational plan. There are many details that must be in place to insure quality patient care, efficient use of office space and resources, and medical-legal protection for the practice. Careful planning can avoid many potential pitfalls. Fundamentally, if sonography is to be part of ones' practice, it must have a high priority. Each practice will identify needs and methods to accomplish these goals.

WHO?

Who will perform the examination? Who will be scanned?

The physician is ultimately responsible for the interpretation of ultrasound studies performed in the office. No office should incorporate sonography into the office practice until there is a physician trained to provide or oversee this service. If the practice hires a sonographer to perform the examination, it is best to hire someone who is a Registered Diagnostic Medical Sonographer (RDMS) or is in the process of registry certification as a measure of adequate training. If an office nurse has undertaken the role of sonographer for a practice without documented training or credentials such as RDMS certification, liability is increased. Remember, however, that the sonographer is not trained to interpret the studies, only in the technical aspects of obtaining them. The sonographer should have clear-cut guidelines for the content of each examination and type of documentation required. There must be some mechanism established for the responsible physician to review the study if he or she is not present during the ultrasound examination. If a physician will be performing the studies, it is critical that adequate time be allotted for this procedure. A hurried examination is worse than no examination at all. At all times during endovaginal sonography, a chaperone should be available regardless of the gender of the provider in order to insure the patient's comfort and to avoid any question of sexual misconduct.

The question of which patients should be scanned is a difficult one. Each obstetric practice must decide whether sonography will be a routine component of prenatal care and, if so, at which gestational age. Some gynecologic practices now incorporate ultrasound as an extension of the bimanual pelvic examination. In contrast, others use ultrasound more selectively. Whichever approach is used, the availability of the equipment, space, and sonographer must meet the needs of the patients and the office routines.

WHEN?

When will patients be scanned?

The indications for the ultrasound examination often will drive the scheduling. For instance, if all patients are to have an ultrasound performed at about 16–20 weeks gestation, it is possible to schedule these in advance. Some practices may choose to designate specified days for these types of procedures, and one or more physician's schedules would be dedicated to these studies. Others may schedule obstetric patients at these gestational ages for an extra 15- to 30-minute visit in order to have dedicated physician- and equipment-time set aside for the studies. It is vital, however, that dedicated time be available for these routine studies. It is difficult and frustrating in the context of a busy schedule to try to perform ultrasound on a PRN (as required) basis without dedicated time. Ultimately, patient care may be affected.

The ultrasound schedule, however, must have enough open time to accommodate the more urgent patient—for instance, the woman with pain and bleeding at 7 weeks gestation or the patient in whom fetal heart tones cannot be auscultated at 34 weeks. It is imperative that quick access to the diagnostic testing be available for them. Importantly, if bad news is obtained from an ultrasound examination, the patient may need extra physician time to help with the news.

WHERE?

Where will the ultrasound machine be kept?

Most practices will have one or two ultrasound machines and these will need to be in dedicated rooms. The rooms must be relatively large to accommodate the patient, the equipment, the provider, the family members, and, perhaps, a chaperone. Ultrasound units produce heat, and adequate ventilation in the room is critical. It is important that the lighting be indirect and physically arranged to prevent both glare on the viewing screen and backlighting behind it. Because the woman's bladder may need to be partially filled for transabdominal scanning and completely empty for transvaginal sonography, it is important that a bathroom be easily available as it may be necessary to use both scanning techniques in the same session.

The issues of patient comfort are easy to address. Although it is possible to scan the patient with her street clothes displaced to reveal her abdomen, care must be taken to avoid smearing her clothing with acoustic coupling gel. Although gel does not stain clothes, it is uncomfortable and messy. Offer the patient the opportunity to change to a patient's gown, provide her with the space to do so as well as a place to hang up her clothes. The acoustic gel is easily warmed by placing the gel bottles in commercially available warming units, baby bottle warmers, or on heating pads. The room should also be equipped with an examination table that will allow the pregnant patient to lie with her head elevated in order to prevent supine hypotension. The examining table should have stirrups to allow for a complete and relatively comfortable transvaginal examination. The equipment should be arranged to allow the patient and her family members to view the screen or (for a relatively modest cost) a secondary monitor may be placed to facilitate viewing.

Occasionally, the ultrasound examination will result in devastating news for the patient. A fetal anomaly may be seen, a fetal death confirmed, or she may have a high likelihood of ovarian cancer based on the findings. An alternate exit that avoids a full waiting room will help preserve the patient's privacy and dignity.

The sonographer's comfort is also important, especially if he or she will be spending long hours performing ultrasound examinations. A comfortable chair is essential and, if the examining table can be electronically controlled, it will diminish the risk of back injury. It is possible, as well, to purchase a large rubber pad to go under the equipment. This provides a comfortable surface on which to stand, and it diminishes the likelihood that an inadvertently dropped transducer will be damaged.

HOW?

How will records be kept? How will scan information get to the patient's chart? How will charges be generated?

Various options for maintaining records of ultrasounds are available, and there are vocal proponents of each. The factors that must be considered include the following: storage space, convenience, hardware requirements, medical-legal advice, type of examination, and cost. Most providers will elect to keep some hard copy of part or all of the examination for a variable period of time. For gynecologic scanning, still pictures recorded either on video tape, paper, or multiformat film (such as is used for radiograph images) may be useful. Recorded images should include documentation of normal anatomy and several images of any pathologic findings. Using the alphanumeric comment feature available on most ultrasound equipment allows for permanent documentation of the findings. For fetal sonography, the same format is available with video, which has the advantage of a dynamic assessment of fetal function that can be recorded.

Hard copy must be clearly identified with some unique system, such as patient name and chart number, as well as the date of the examination. Individual print pictures could be filed in the patient's office chart or in a separate ultrasound chart. Use of multiformat images requires separate camera developers and filing systems. Many patient scans can be recorded on a single 120 minute VHS tape, although the shelf-life of a VHS tape may not be much more than 5–7 years. The storage of VHS tape is surprisingly easy. If video taping is used, a complete log of each patient seen must be maintained, so that the study can be easily retrieved and reviewed as needed.

A written summary of the findings should be included in the patient's chart. This could be handwritten in the office chart or dictated, depending on the resources available. It is important that results that directly affect patient care be available as they are needed. Do not rely merely on memory but clearly document the interpretation and objective findings.

As a medical procedure, sonography appears in the *Current Procedural Terminology* (CPT) book, and procedure codes should be submitted to reimbursement agencies accurately describing what procedure you performed. Familiarity with the complexities of CPT coding, which can change from year to year, is critical to insure accurate reporting and appropriate reimbursement for services rendered.

WHAT?

What type of equipment should be used?

Contemporary, commercially available ultrasound units range from simple to extremely complex models, and most vendors offer a complete range. The most critical step is to have a clear sense of what type of equipment and special features are important for your practice and what you don't need. Before purchasing or leasing equipment, call many of the vendors. Most manufacturers will bring a demonstration model to your practice with an applications specialist and will allow potential buyers to use the equipment for a short while. Shop around and compare the different products. Critically appraise not only the image quality in your patients but also the ease of use of the equipment. Is the software reasonable? Are there options to add biometric charts that you want to use? Is it easy to change probes? Are there options missing that are important to you, such as a cine loop, Doppler, editing features, split screen, twins package? Are there too many features on the equipment? Can you use a simpler model? What are the cost and content of the service contract? It is important to ask the sales representative for names of other users of the equipment in similar practices so that you can get an opinion from another user.

SUMMARY

Each practice will develop a unique way to incorporate ultrasound. The same issues, however, apply to wherever ultrasound is used: the labor and delivery unit, emergency department, and in-patient units. It is important to plan in advance, so that patient care is optimal and so that ultrasound does not become the tail that wags the dog.

20

Origins and Control of Liability in Obstetrical and Gynecological Ultrasound

Few experiences produce anxiety comparable to that provoked by the role of defendant in a legal action to recover damages from medical negligence. Most medical practitioners believe they provide, at all times, the best service possible and are angry, hurt, and defensive when faced with malpractice action or when accused of negligence. All clinical services are possible sources of allegations of professional negligence and consequent actions to recover damages.

The medical practitioner must at all times and under all circumstances endeavor to provide the most appropriate possible service to the patient. Unfortunately, even with the best care, adverse outcomes occur that, with reasonable examination, are beyond anyone's control. Therefore, the practitioner active in ob/gyn ultrasound does undertake a degree of medical liability in the provision of that service. Obstetrical and gynecological ultrasound is neither immune to nor uniquely vulnerable to allegations of negligence. There are, however, specific efforts that may minimize, but cannot eliminate, the risk of malpractice litigation arising from ob/gyn ultrasound.

TORT LAW

Successful legal action to recover damages, or relieve the plaintiff of the economic burden of those damages, requires that certain facts be established in evidence. The specific definition of these requirements varies from state to state, but general similarities are found. Each of these elements of a malpractice litigation must be established in fact, and, in individual situations, any of these may be challenged and represent a basis for successful defense. First, a relationship between the patient and the physician is required; second, medical care that falls below the standard of care is necessary; third, damages must be documented; and, finally, the negligence in evidence must have caused the damages.

281

A professional relationship is necessary to establish an obligation, or duty, on the part of the physician to provide appropriate care. Generally, a professional license to practice, a professional place of business, an established account or medical file for the patient, or specific assignment of the physician defendant to a professional activity within an institution in which the patient has an established relationship or establishes a relationship by virtue of presentation for care at that institution are sufficient to establish the necessary basis for the obligation or duty to provide adequate or standard services.

The plaintiff must show that the care provided fell below the standard of care. The exact definition of *standard of care* varies among the states, but generally it is that care that would have been provided by any reasonable practitioner with similar training in that community when presented with similar circumstances. The standard of care, then, may vary or at least be open to debate. Clearly, there are examples of negligence that support little discussion or debate. The administration of an incorrect medication or surgery performed on the wrong knee are possible events that are difficult to justify. However, the quality of the relationship, the true nature of any damages, or the causitive relationship of the negligent act, and the damages may be open to question.

Clinical care, however, is rarely so straightforward and simple. Subjective interpretation, perception, and educated speculation are often inherent elements of medical service. Medical care is typically provided within a range of possibilities for the diagnosis and the intervention intended to alleviate the condition. The plaintiff must show that, under the circumstances of the care in question, the defendant provided substandard care. To establish this fact, experts are employed to examine the medical record and the testimony of relevant witnesses and to render an opinion regarding the quality of the care provided. Is a subspecialist in a tertiery referral center held to the same standard as a general practitioner or to a standard established for subspecialists?

The primary sources of evidence are the medical record and the memories of witnesses. Often, the events took place years before the court action. Although the defendant's memory of events may be biased against the plaintiff, clearly the defendant's memory may be biased against the plaintiff. Therefore, nonaligned witnesses and the medical record provide important sources of evidence. If events, observations, considerations, decisions, or alternatives are not well described in the record, the effect is as if they never happened. If a complex clinical event is well described, the observations of the physician clearly spelled out, the diagnostic, and therapeutic alternatives clearly considered, and the basis for a specific diagnosis and treatment explained, then the debate becomes an examination of the physician's judgment, and it becomes far more difficult to prove negligence. If, however, the medical record is poor, with little in the way of explanation or discussion, the allegation of negligence is easier to propose. Despite the defendant's clear memory of his or her thinking or the reasons for a particular choice, without a record, the plaintiff may allege that the examination was incomplete, the assessment was shallow and shoddy, and no therapeutic alternatives were considered. A poor medical record is an open invitation to an allegation of negligence.

Damages must be established, and they may be real, general, or special. Real damages are direct costs related to the negligent act such as further surgery, extended care, or other services necessary to restore the patient to his or her prior condition. General damages, consequential to the negligent act, such as lost income, anxiety, or mental trauma, may require the testimony of professional experts as to the degree of trauma or the estimated earning potential of the victim of the negligence. Special damages, or punitive damages, are to punish the defendant for the negligence.

The negligence must have caused the damages. Coincidental negligence that is not related to the damages in evidence is not a basis for recovery. The plaintiff must establish that the alleged negligence did, in fact, cause the damages. All other elements of a case established in fact, a challenge of causation may be the basis for a successful defense.

In civil litigation, the plaintiff is required to establish in evidence only that the negligent act more likely than not caused the damages. This degree of certainty at its minimum is only 51% probability, not the criminal standard of "beyond reasonable doubt." There was or there was not a relationship. There were or there were not damages. The defendant is or is not guilty of a substandard or negligent act or service. These elements may be argued and challenged but, in the end, the jury or judge must reach a conclusion one way or the other. However, in the case of causation, the verdict may favor the plaintiff with 49% acknowledged uncertainty remaining.

The art of argument and the communication skills of the defendant, the plaintiffs, and the expert witnesses for both sides clearly affect the outcome of any civil legal action. Cases may or may not be decided exclusively on the basis of undisputed facts in evidence. Legal action typically takes years to reach resolution, regardless of the nature of that resolution. The anger and pain in both the plaintiffs and the defendants is unrelieved until the conflict is finally resolved. Any measures directed at promoting optimal services, avoiding misunderstandings, and preventing legal action is more than worth the effort.

NEGLIGENCE AND LAWSUITS

Most negligence does not result in legal action. Most legal action does not result from negligence. A recent review of medical records of a large New England medical center to identify objectively negligent acts that resulted in adverse outcomes found that few of these events resulted in legal action. Furthermore, during the same period, few of the legal actions initiated against care provided in that same center resulted from acts that had been identified prospectively by the investigators as negligent.

The features of a clinical relationship, then, that contribute to the initiation of legal action, go beyond the obvious events of care. The quality of communication, the patient's understanding of the goals and limits of treatment, and the attitude of the professionals are often identified as more important in the birth of a lawsuit than the clinical events themselves. Subjective liability, therefore, is increased by poor communication resulting in unrealistic goals and expectations on the part of the patient. If a patient who leaves the office after hearing that "the baby is fine" believes she has been given a guarantee against any unexpected malformation or adverse outcome, she might feel cheated with any other outcome and inquire of an attorney whether she has a basis for action. Win or lose, such action causes years of anxiety and misery. Winning or losing may hinge on the adequacy of the medical records, the quality of documentation of training and background in ultrasound, and the skills of the expert witnesses.

Is a reasonable effort to produce reasonable and realistic expectations in the patient an option to minimize these sorts of misunderstandings and potential liability? You bet!

LIABILITY IN ULTRASOUND

Medical liability in ultrasound arises primarily from three sources including failure to use the technique when indicated, failure to perform a standard service, and failure to properly interpret the information.

Failure to Use Ultrasound When Indicated

Indications for ob/gyn ultrasound are many, varied, and expanding daily. The National Institutes of Health convened a Consensus Development Conference in 1984 that published a document that concluded that routine use of ultrasound in obstetrics could not at that time be supported by the available literature. That document did offer 28 indications for obstetrical ultrasound that remain recognized standards (see Table 4-1, page 44).

Alleged negligence may take the form of failure of the responsible physician or provider to respond to reasonable clinical evidence of one or more of these circumstances with an ultrasound examination followed by an adverse outcome. For instance, during the course of prenatal care, measurement of the uterus is standard practice. If the fundal height is found to be 32 cm at 26 weeks gestation, but an ultrasound examination is not considered to resolve this apparent discrepancy and an adverse outcome such as premature birth of twins or perinatal complication associated with an unexpected twin birth is documented, the failure to use the technique in response to reasonable evidence of a problem may be the basis for legal action. Another example involves the late registrant. If a patient registers after 20-weeks gestation and/or is unsure of the date of her last menstrual period but ultrasound is not requested to establish gestational age, and later a complication of pregnancy or adverse outcome is suffered that might have been prevented or better treated if accurate gestational age were known, such damages might form the basis of legal action.

Another failure to use ultrasound that has contributed to the allegation of negligence is failure to estimate fetal weight in the case of a pregnancy at risk for fetal macrosomia with subsequent perinatal birth trauma. Although the accuracy and precision of sonographic estimation of fetal weight is limited, failure to recognize risk factors for fetal macrosomia such as maternal obesity, gestational diabetes, excessive maternal weight gain, or prior birth of a macrosomia infant, may form the basis for the allegation of negligence.

Indications for ultrasound in gynecology are less-well established. Ultrasound is one of several imaging techniques that may be useful to the gynecologist in the evaluation of dysfunction or disease, including magnetic resonance imaging, and radiographic techniques, including hysterosalpingography. Therefore, ultrasound does not enjoy the same unique utility in gynecology that it does in obstetrics, although certain specific clinical applications are generally recognized as helpful, including

- examination of adnexal mass
- evaluation of uterine myomata
- assessment of pelvic pain
- assessment of postpartum hemorrhage
- monitor ovulation induction.

The routine screening of perimenopausal and postmenopausal patients for ovarian or endometrial disease is the topic of investigation and interest but yet of unproved value.

FAILURE TO PERFORM A STANDARD SERVICE

Alleged failure to perform a standard obstetrical ultrasound examination is a common basis for liability. Sustaining such an allegation requires that the plaintiff establish the standard of care for an ultrasound examination and to prove that the service provided fell below that standard.

The American College of Obstetricians and Gynecologists (ACOG) published guidelines for obstetrical ultrasound examination in Technical Bulletin #139, in 1993. Furthermore, the American College of Radiologists (ACR) and the American Institute of Ultrasound in Medicine (AIUM) together published guidelines for content of the obstetrical ultrasound examination in 1986, and updated the guidelines in 1991. These two sources of standards do not agree completely, but there are many similarities and only a few differences (see Table 4-4, page 48).

First, the differences. The ACOG's guidelines recognize two levels of obstetrical ultrasound, basic and targeted (comprehensive). The basic examination might be one performed in the generalist's office on the patient not known to be at risk for any specific fetal problem, and the targeted is intended to specifically search for a fetal problem suspected to exist. This regionalized concept is not different from the regionalization that characterizes most other medical services, but it does assume that the provider is providing a good faith effort to assess risk for fetal abnormalities in his or her patients. A reasonable attempt to assess risk factors for congenital disease or malformation is necessary to justify performing ultrasound on low-risk patients.

The ACR/AIUM guidelines do not define two levels of ultrasound but specify minimum content recommended for all such examinations. This assumes equal skill, training, and background for all practitioners, a concept that is questionable. The other major difference between the two sets of guidelines is documentation. The ACOG does not discuss the nature or quality of the documentation of the ultrasound examination. ACR/AIUM does specify the images recommended and that images be recorded that document the findings.

The similarities of the two sets of guidelines are striking, and they form the basis for the rest of the discussion.

OBSTETRICAL ULTRASOUND MINIMUM CONTENT

The obstetrical ultrasound examination should consist of three categories of information: a survey of uterine contents, fetal biometry, and a fetal anatomic screening examination (see sample report form).

Survey

Uterine contents should be assessed, including fetal number (Fig. 20-1), position (Fig. 20-2), viability, amniotic fluid volume (Fig. 20-3), placental location, and an assessment of the adnexae.

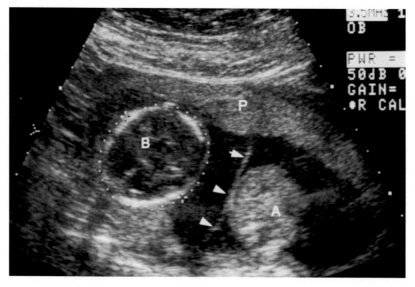

FIG. 20-1. The uterine survey shown here documents twins separated by a membrane. The membrane is not a casual observation and should be recorded in the report.

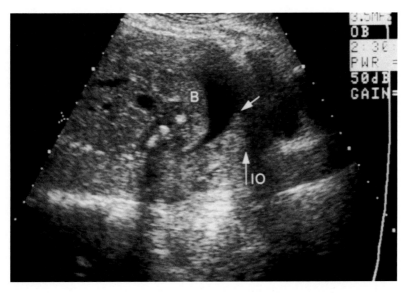

FIG. 20-2. Fetal malpresentation is often associated with abnormal placentation as illustrated here. The internal os of the cervix *(IO)* is overlain by this posterior placenta previa *(arrows)*. The breech is seen above *(B)*.

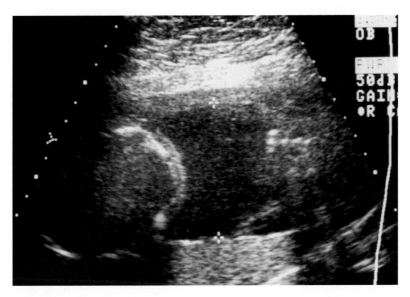

FIG. 20-3. Assessment and documentation of amniotic fluid is illustrated here. Amniotic fluid may be assessed subjectively, although in the extremes of oligohydramnios and polyhydramnios some semiobjective assessment is helpful. Here, a single vertical dimension is recorded.

Biometry

Fetal biometry should include crown-rump length if appropriate, or biparietal diameter or head circumference, abdominal circumference, and femur length. Discrepancies in estimated gestational age should be addressed. The first response to a discrepancy is to repeat the measurement, the second is to assess relevant anatomy to evaluate the possibility that an anomaly has caused the asymmetrical growth, and finally to reach some conclusion regarding a persistent asymmetry.

Fetal Anatomic Screen

Fetal anatomy should be thoroughly reviewed, including craniospinal, thoracic and cardiac, abdominal and urinary tract, and skeletal anatomy. Recommended minimum image planes include

- Cranial occipito-frontal [standard biparietal diameter (BPD)] (Fig. 20-4)
- Cranial suboccipito-bregmatic (posterior fossa)
- Spine coronal longitudinal (2–3 views) (Fig. 20-5)
- Four-chamber heart (Fig. 20-6)

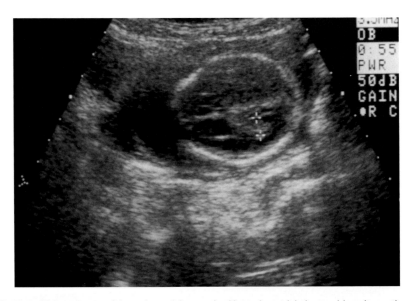

FIG. 20-4. Measurement of the atrium of the cerebral lateral ventricle is considered a routine assessment. If the choroid fills the atrium, measurement is not necessary. However, if cerebrospinal fluid separates the choroid from the medial wall, measurement is recommended. Measured perpendicular to the axis of the ventricle, not to include the walls, the diameter should not exceed 10 mm.

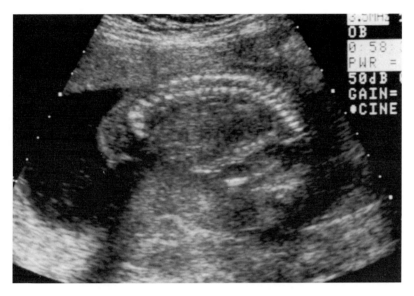

FIG. 20-5. As discussed in Chapter 10, this oblique longitudinal view of the fetal spine is visually appealing and includes most of the ventrally flexed spine in a single plane, but it is the least sensitive for small dysraphic lesions compared with sequential coronal views.

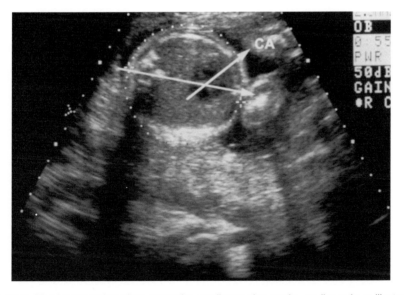

FIG. 20-6. The four-chamber view, assessing cardiac-to-chest ratio, cardiac axis as illustrated here should intersect *(crossed arrows)* the sagittal midline at about 45 degrees.

- Transverse abdomen with stomach (Fig. 20-7)
- Transverse abdomen at cord insertion (Fig. 20-8A,B)
- Kidneys and bladder
- Femur (one or both) (Fig. 20-9)

The detail available from a realtime ultrasound examination is great. The anatomic screening images listed above are the minimum appropriate in the case of a pregnancy not known to be at risk for a fetal abnormality. If any historical or clinical risk factor for fetal abnormality is known, more extensive examination is indicated, and consideration of referral to an individual with the training and experience required to provide maximum diagnostic accuracy is recommended. Furthermore, if, in the course of this low-risk or basic examination, a desired image cannot be produced or appears unusual in any way, referral for a second opinion is appropriate. Failure to ask for a second opinion under such circumstances would likely increase liability in the event of an adverse outcome.

Gynecological Content

The presence or absence, shape, size, and consistency of the uterus, the location, size, and appearance of the adnexae, and the contents of the cul-de-sac form the basic elements of the gynecological ultrasound examination. The thickness of the endometrium should be recorded as well.

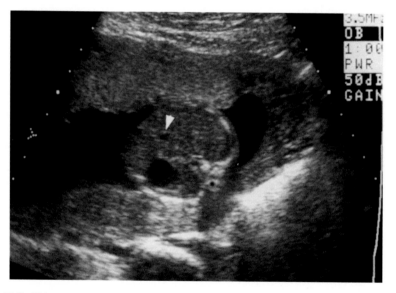

FIG. 20-7. This transverse sonogram at the level of the stomach and umbilical vein *(arrowhead)* also includes thoracic spine and kidneys.

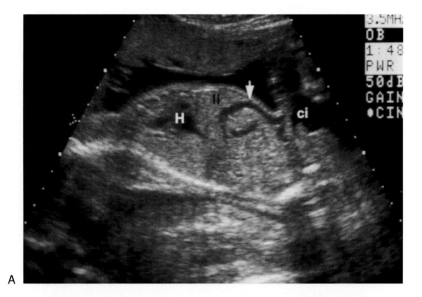

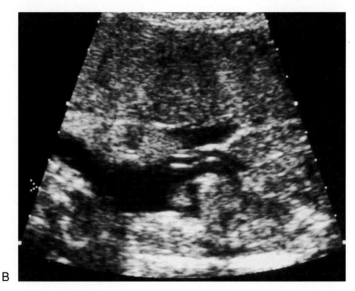

FIG. 20-8A. This sagittal view shows heart in the chest *(H)*, umbilical vein for virtually its entire intrafetal length *(arrow)*, and the cord insertion in the lower abdomen *(ci)*. *li,* liver. **B:** The cord insertion viewed in transverse plane shows an abrupt entry in the lower abdominal midline. Omphalocele and gastroschisis are virtually excluded by this view.

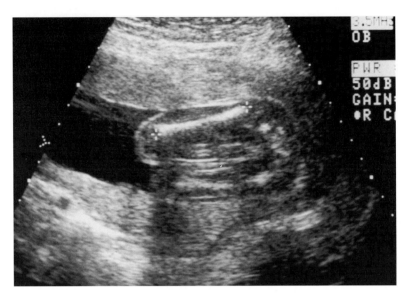

FIG. 20-9. At least one femur is recommended as a screening in the case of the patient not known to be at increased risk for a short limb dysplasia as seen here.

If ovarian masses or cysts are noted, they should be individually measured and their structural characteristics, described. Large myomata may be measured for future comparison.

ABBREVIATED ULTRASOUND EXAMINATIONS

Although recent ACOG Committee Opinion supports a number of clinical circumstances that allow the performance of an abbreviated obstetrical ultrasound examination, liability for missed diagnoses or inappropriate interventions resulting from abbreviated examinations is increased. The brief ultrasound examination upon admission to labor and delivery with a suspected malpresentation simply to confirm the presentation cannot, in most circumstances, be justified. If a clinician just "takes a peek to be sure it's a breech," then performs a cesarean delivery of an anencephalic infant, the potential liability is obvious. Malformation is a major cause of malpresentation and should be excluded in any case of malpresentation prior to operative delivery. In only three types of clinical circumstance might any abbreviated examination be defended.

First, emergent events prevent the performance of a complete examination. The examination is performed in a labor and delivery unit and simultaneous events clearly require immediate attention and prevent a complete examination. Perhaps the patient being examined is experiencing rapidly progressive labor, or other patients are in the process of emergent events that require the provider's attention. If emergent circumstances are the basis for an abbreviated examination and reasonable efforts to obtain a complete examination by some other means are not likely to be successful, the circumstances should be documented in the record.

Second, maternal habitus or fetal position prevents adequate images of a standard anatomic area. Obesity imposes acoustic artifacts that often obscure fetal soft tissue detail and prevent sensitive examination. Deep pelvic engagement of the fetal vertex may prevent sensitive examination of internal, soft tissue anatomy. Overlaying twins may obscure the anatomy of the deeper twin. If any of these circumstances prevent adequate visualization of important anatomy, this problem should be documented in the record.

Third, the patient may have undergone a complete ultrasound examination during this pregnancy by the provider or another sonologist or sonographer with whom the practitioner is familiar and whose quality of examination satisfies him or her. Even so, the practitioner takes some risk that the prior examination missed important diagnostic information or that a fetal abnormality that may not have been apparent at that earlier examination would now be apparent and would influence clinical management.

FAILURE TO INTERPRET APPROPRIATELY

Misinterpretation of ultrasound images, misdiagnosis of twins, or failed diagnosis of twins or triplets does increase liability risk. The production of defective biometric measurements and the assumption that the estimated gestational age is accurate may lead to delivery interventions at inappropriate times with adverse consequences. Such circumstances result in a liability burden. It is, therefore, incumbent upon the provider engaged in obstetrical ultrasound to pursue the necessary training and regular updates and to endeavor to provide accurate and appropriate services. The active performance of obstetrical ultrasound without any evidence of prior training or supervision or sustained efforts to improve skills obviously results in increased liability in the event of any adverse outcome related to these services.

LIABILITY CONTROL IN OB/GYN ULTRASOUND

There are three ways in which a practitioner can control the liability associated with obstetrical or gynecological ultrasound: he or she can 1. provide a standard of care service; 2. document the service provided; and 3. educate the patient about the reasonable goals and limitations of the service. The *primary* issue is the provision of a high-quality service, and, when service of the highest quality is provided, although adverse outcomes will unfortunately still occur, liability associated with the ultrasound examination will be minimized. Documentation and patient education are secondary efforts that can diminish but not eliminate the probability of legal action.

Optimal Service

Do your homework. Document the level of training you received in your residency program and retain that documentation. The time is coming when hospital or third-party-payer accreditation for privileges or payment may require documentation. Keep records of your postgraduate courses that are relevant to ultrasound and consider keeping a journal of personal ultrasound experience at least for a period of months to establish the level of your practice skills. Discuss and establish the expected content of every ultrasound examination performed in your practice and establish some guidelines for referral so that every member of the practice is held to the same guidelines.

Never make a mistake. Although this seems an unreasonable expectation, it is, nonetheless, a serious goal to provide the best possible service by following an agreed-upon set of guidelines that generally follow the nationally recognized guidelines outlined above in a methodical manner. It is not necessary to mimic either set of guidelines exactly, but any major exception should be carefully considered.

A dedicated office examination form that provides a check box or space for each major feature of the examination would serve not only as a report form but also as a guide to the performance of a complete examination. Do not adopt a form with a lot of boxes or spaces that will be left empty. Do produce a form that everyone in the practice can live with and can agree to. Do follow the form.

In the case of images that do not appear exactly as expected or cannot be made to appear normal, do not pass them off as the result of having a bad day. Suspect the possibility, but only the possibility, of an abnormality. A good working relationship with a referral facility should be established and used. Do not hesitate to ask for a second opinion in every case that looks suspicious. Expect feedback from your referral resource and find alternative backup if you do not get regular feedback. You should expect to learn from most referrals, whether they turn out to be normal or not. The identification and use of a good referral resource is part of an optimal service.

Documentation

Document the performance of a standard-of-care service. Documentation may serve as a clinical resource for future management decisions, a research database, or as a way to show that a standard-of-care service was performed. Documentation of clinical services may take many forms including a chart note, a dedicated office form, multiple still pictures in a variety of formats, or videotape. The type of documentation varies and is not the subject of recognized guidelines. Because ultrasound is an examination based in images, a chart note alone or even a dedicated form alone, although useful in promoting the performance of a complete examination, are not considered sufficient documentation. Still photos, whether paper, photographic, or digital format are limited as well. No matter how many still photographs are produced, they are a poor substitute for the many minutes of realtime images that constituted the examination. At a minimum, a photograph of each of the standard biometric measures, amniotic fluid, and each of the anatomic screening images is recommended.

Videotape of the uterine survey, the biometry, and the fetal anatomic survey is the most complete documentation of the examination available. Videotape equipment is relatively inexpensive, and a large number of examinations may be saved for years on each long-play tape. Storage and indexing are not difficult or burdensome. Broadcast quality video is not required to show that a standard service was provided. Certainly, it is possible that videotape may document a misdiagnosis or failed diagnosis. However, many more cases will be successfully defended than lost by the documentation of a standard service. It is easier to argue that total diagnostic sensitivity is not and cannot be expected in the basic ultrasound examination of a low-risk patient if a standard examination is documented than it is to defend the negligence of not having performed or not having documented a standard examination.

Patient Education

Recall that the majority of legal actions do not result from objective negligence. The majority of patients will not initiate legal action regardless of culpability. A small minority of patients will initiate legal action regardless of innocence. Between these extremes are patients who might consider litigation in the case of an adverse outcome if they feel cheated or wronged. Patient expectations play an important role in the subjective perception of negligence and in the likelihood of litigation.

An effort to limit expectations to reasonable goals and to educate the patient is worth the time in order to reduce the probability of misperceptions and unrealistic expectations. Remember, the outcome of litigation turns on many subjective points including communication skills, believability of witnesses, quality and detail of the medical record, and persuasiveness of expert testimony. Win or lose, a lawsuit causes years of misery for both plaintiff and defendant. Reasonable expectations are well worth any effort it takes to produce them.

Written, informed consent may or may not suit your practice. Consider a form such as the example provided. A brief attempt to address issues of indication, safety, and limits of service in plain language and with obvious concern for patient welfare will help limit expectations. Answer any questions that arise in an open and honest manner. Talk to the patient during the examination. Interaction during the examination has been shown to reduce patient anxiety. Do not promise

ULTRASOUND REPORT FORM

Patient Name_____

Medical Record#_____Date_____

Clinical Indication_____

EDC_____Clinical EGA_____

Uterine Survey:

Fetal Number _____

Viability   Y   N

Position   Cephalic   __
           Breech   __
           Transverse   __
           Oblique   __

Amniotic Fluid   Normal   __
               Increased   __
               Decreased   __
               AFI(cm)   __

Placenta   Anterior   __
           Posterior   __
           Fundal   __
           Low   __
           Previa   __

Fetal Biometry:

BPD   _____mm   _____wks

HC   _____mm   _____wks

AC   _____mm   _____wks

FL   _____mm   _____wks

AVG US EGA   _____wks

US EFW   _____g

Range of EFW +/−   _____g

Fetal Anatomic Screen:

    Cranial contour   _____

    Lateral ventricles   _____

    Posterior fossa   _____

    Spine   _____

    Four chamber   _____

    Stomach   _____

    Umbilicus   _____

    Kidneys   _____

    Bladder   _____

    Limbs   _____

Comments:

_____

_____

_____

_____

_____

_____

_____

_____

_____

_____

Biophysical Observations:

Trunk   Y   N   Limb   Y   N

FBM   Y   N   AFI>5   Y   N   Score _____

Comments:_____

_____

_____

_____

Examiner_____   Videotape: Y   N #_____

OBSTETRICAL ULTRASOUND

It has been recommended that you undergo an ultrasound examination. Obstetrical ultrasound is a method of producing images of the baby using short pulses of very high pitched sound. These pulses of sound are reflected as echoes by body parts and the echoes are detected and used to construct the pictures. There is no known danger to the baby from these pulses of sound in spite of extensive research directed at detecting any such danger. However, though ultrasound seems to be safe, it is not wise to overdo the examination since we can never be completely sure that some side effect will not ever be discovered in the future. Therefore, although family members are welcome, do not ask for extended unnecessary scanning for their enjoyment alone.

The recommendation for this examination comes from questions about your pregnancy and the knowledge that ultrasound can tell us about how far along your pregnancy is, whether or not you carry twins, whether there is enough fluid around your baby, how well the baby is growing, whether the baby is head down or not, and where the placenta, or afterbirth, is located inside the womb. This is information that can significantly help your doctor take better care of you and your baby.

If there were any reason to suspect the possibility of a birth defect, such as a family history of a baby with a birth defect, or an abnormal screening test result, you may be referred to a center for an ultrasound examination specifically looking for that defect. Ultrasound in general is not capable of eliminating the possibility of a birth defect, and this examination is not specifically targeting birth defects because your baby is not considered to be at high risk for a malformation. Unfortunately, however, birth defects can occur without any reasons for suspicion. Therefore, even if today's examination is perfectly normal, we cannot give you a guarantee of a perfectly normal baby.

We will ask you to sign this page only to show that we discussed these ideas with you and that you had the chance to read and question this information and give your permission for the examination. If you have questions, please ask them now. We understand that you expect us to do our very best to produce complete, accurate, and useful information for you and for your doctor.

_____   _____
Patient   Spouse

_____   _____
Witness   Date

what you cannot deliver. Do not be careless with comments about how normal the baby is, although it is perfectly acceptable to say that, to the best of your ability, you have determined that everything you examined appeared normal. Do say that you cannot offer a guarantee of a normal outcome.

SUMMARY

Be methodical. Follow recognized standards and do not perform abbreviated examinations except under specific documented circumstances. Document the provision of a standard examination in both written and image form using the format that you feel suits your practice and circumstances. Inform the patient in simple but adequate terms about the reasonable goals and limits of the examination. Do not promise what you cannot deliver. Deliver the best service possible.

FURTHER READING

Diagnostic Ultrasound Imaging in Pregnancy. Published by The Department of Health and Human Services. February, 1984. Available from U.S. Government Printing Office, Washington, D.C. 20402.

Guidelines for Performance of the Antepartum Obstetrical Ultrasound Examination. American Institute of Ultrasound in Medicine.

Perone N, Carpenter RJ, Robertson JA. Legal liability in the use of ultrasound by office based obstetricians. *Am J Obstet Gynecol* 1984;150:801.

Ultrasound Imaging in Pregnancy. ACOG Committee Opinion #96, August, 1991. Committee on Obstetrics: Maternal and Fetal Medicine, ACOG, Washington, D.C. (Replaced by ACOG Technical Bulletin #187, December, 1993.)

Ultrasonography in Pregnancy. ACOG Technical Bulletin #187, December, 1993. ACOG Resource Center, 409 12th Street, S.W., Washington, D.C.

Subject Index

Note: Page numbers in *italic* type indicate figures, tables, and illustrations.